MINDING EMOTIONS

Psychoanalysis and Psychological Science

Elliot Jurist, *Series Editor*

Books in this series aim to bridge the work of researchers and the work of clinicians. They reflect the current empirical findings and state of the art in psychoanalysis and psychodynamic treatment. They are written to be practical and relevant to clinicians.

**Attachment and Psychoanalysis:
Theory, Research, and Clinical Implications**
Morris N. Eagle

**Minding Emotions:
Cultivating Mentalization in Psychotherapy**
Elliot Jurist

MINDING EMOTIONS

Cultivating Mentalization
in Psychotherapy

ELLIOT JURIST

THE GUILFORD PRESS
New York   London

Library of Congress Cataloging-in-Publication Data

Names: Jurist, Elliot L., 1953– author.
Title: Minding emotions : cultivating mentalization in psychotherapy / Elliot
    Jurist.
Description: New York : Guilford Press, [2018] | Series: Psychoanalysis and
    psychological science | Includes bibliographical references and index.
Identifiers: LCCN 2017037597 | ISBN 9781462534999 (hardcover) |
    ISBN 9781462542918 (paperback)
Subjects: LCSH: Emotions. | Psychotherapy. | Mentalization Based Therapy.
Classification: LCC RC489.E45 .J87 2018 | DDC 616.89/14—dc23
LC record available at *https://lccn.loc.gov/2017037597*

For Rebecca, Julia, and Joshua
so much

About the Author

Elliot Jurist, PhD, is Professor of Psychology and Philosophy at The Graduate Center, The City University of New York, where he served as Director of the Clinical Psychology Doctoral Program from 2004 to 2013. His research focuses on mentalization and the role of emotions in psychotherapy. Dr. Jurist is the coauthor of *Affect Regulation, Mentalization, and the Development of the Self*; and coeditor of *Mind to Mind: Infant Research, Neuroscience, and Psychoanalysis.* He is also the editor of the Guilford book series Psychoanalysis and Psychological Science and the editor of *Psychoanalytic Psychology*, the journal of Division 39 (Psychoanalysis) of the American Psychological Association. He is a recipient of the Scholarship Award from Division 39, among other honors.

Preface

As I write this preface, I am imagining a kinship with the many authors who feel the weight of having begun their work at one point in time and ending in what seems like a completely different era. Words do not come easily to register the gruesomeness of this time—the utter stupidity, the transparent crudeness, the revolting gloating, the orchestration and threat of violence, and the steady parade of dishonesty and lies that define our president and the current regime in the United States of America.

Can a book on emotions overlook this? Is it possible to rise above outrage—the shock and anger at the enormous, unnecessary suffering of our fellow human beings who, as immigrants and refugees, risk being literally without a home? Is it possible to push aside the profound sense of mourning—the enveloping sadness that democracy, however imperfectly realized, could turn out to be so vulnerable? No, no, and no.

There is good reason to fear the unleashing of emotions and good reason to believe that we need to tend to them now more than ever. This book welcomes emotions in all of their complexity—how they manifest themselves (for better and worse) in everyday life, and especially in psychotherapy, and how we might cultivate their use without overestimating our ability to fathom them. The project is perhaps best characterized by the aspiration "to do things with emotions." I begin by recognizing a category of not knowing what we feel, what I term "aporetic emotions," and I end by featuring the idea of "mentalized affectivity," the capacity to reflect on emotions in light of autobiographical memory. The book is interdisciplinary in scope, mixing theory, research, clinical work, and autobiographical memoir—an attempt to render psychoanalytic ideas relevant for the present and to thrive more broadly into the future. Along the way, I express reservations about current notions of "emotional intelligence" and "emotion regulation," both of which, perhaps not by intention but by consequence, serve to reward the privileged. I am dubious of our capacity to control our emotions, and especially wish to reject the miserable assumption that unregulated emotions are, by definition, undesirable and unhealthy.

A crucial argument that I make in Chapter 6 is that mentalized affectivity defines what makes psychotherapy work, and that all psychotherapy can be construed as an attempt to improve communication. Communication is an evolutionary concept, akin to other biological instincts, and at the same time is strongly influenced and informed by culture. It has a distinct connotation from the hortatory, everyday sense of the term. Ultimately, I propose that communication in psychotherapy relies on epistemic trust, epistemic circumspection, and truthfulness. If truthfulness motivates and brings the therapeutic process to fruition, the implications of life outside of and beyond therapy must be at stake, hence the inescapability that psychotherapy must be implicated in our current political morass.

Can the institution of psychotherapy survive in a culture where truthfulness is not valued and perhaps coded as a loser strategy, a waste of time that could be otherwise wasted? It remains to be seen. It also remains to be seen whether the institution of psychotherapy might rejuvenate itself, refusing the conceit that truthfulness is a value of private life alone. My hope in any case is to support the attempt to rethink and reimagine psychotherapy as a place to know what one feels and to live with the consequences (which in no way is meant to connote passivity).

A premise of my book is that emotions and emotion regulation are deeply and inevitably social. This does not have to limit us to a contagion of conformism. Indeed, my hope is that this book will be read as falling on the side of resistance. Resistance in politics has almost the opposite meaning to resistance in mental health, as a patient once commented to me. Let us strive not to miss the healthy side of resistance in therapy and to celebrate the potential for therapists and patients to embrace a new spirit of agency—ready and able to struggle against the powers that be.

I wish to thank Nat Sufrin for his sharp eye in completing the references and Jonela Kolasi for her help with the tables. Special thanks to David Greenberg, lead author on the Mentalized Affectivity Scale, included here in the Appendix (and thanks to Camilla Hegsted and Yoni Berkowitz, who also worked on the creation of the scale and the 2017 article).

I also wish to thank students, colleagues, and friends for conversation and feedback: Julie Ackerman, Nancy Adler, Jon Allen, Liz Allison, Stephen Anen, Ken Barish, Karin Belser, Dickon Bevington, Efrain

Bleiberg, Phil Blumberg, Jane Caflisch, Chris Christian, Liat Claridge, Ricardo Corbetta, Diana Diamond, Morris Eagle, Eric Fertuck, Peter Fonagy, Arthur Fox, Kobe Frances, Wendy Carolina Franco, Roger Frie, Dana Fuchs, Mark Gerald, Bill Gottdiener, Libby Graf, Monica Grandy, Sibel Halfon, Jaleh Hamadani, Ben Harris, Loryn Hatch, Yianna Ioannou, Teresa Lopez-Castro, Patrick Luyten, Johanna Malone, Bill MacGillivray, Alice Mangan, Kevin Meehan, Nancy McWilliams, Catherine Monk, Marley Oakes, Spiros Orfanos, Ian Pervil, Remy Potier, Olga Poznansky, Diana Puñales, Olivier Putois, Andrea Recarte, Joseph Reynoso, Margaret Rosario, Arielle Rubinstein, Sasha Rudenstine, Jeremy Safran, Banu Seckin, Henry Seiden, Carla Sharp, Neil Skolnick, Tzachi Slonim, Mary Target, Steve Tuber, Paul Wachtel, Tempe Watts, Joel Weinberger, Josh Weinstein, Lissa Weinstein, Lutz Wittmann, Lisa Wolfe, and Lauren Young. I would also like to express my gratitude to my friends Cliff Simms and György Gergely, both of whom have sustained me with over 35 years of animated intellectual and political discussions—may they continue!

It is a pleasure to recognize the support and love that I have received from my family: Sumner Jurist, Andra Jurist and Bruce Stewart, Lindsay Jurist-Rosner, Marney Jurist-Rosner, Judy and Len Wharton, Ruth and Stephen McDonald, Ben McDonald, Andrew McDonald, Nat Wharton and Sophie Faure-Wharton, and Sasha Wharton—and also Ralph Wharton, Stephanie Bernheim, and Naida Wharton. I feel fortunate to be part of this extended family. To my wife, Rebecca Wharton, and my children, Joshua and Julia: thank you for supporting me in the relatively selfish enterprise of waking up early and isolating myself to work, but for also refusing to grant me too much liberty in that direction! Rebecca's labor kept us afloat and nurtured us all, and I treasure the love that prevails in our lives. I would be remiss to forget the dogs, beloved Sonia and Pretzel, who contributed mightily with their periodic but regular demands for us to be restored with fresh air in Riverside Park.

Finally, I wish to thank Jim Nageotte of The Guilford Press, whose fine eye absolutely and categorically made this a better book (even if he might have preferred just one adverb here), and Seymour Weingarten, with whom I have enjoyed conversation over many years. Seymour is a towering figure in the world of psychology, and, in particular, psychoanalytic publishing, and his contribution deserves our abiding gratitude.

Contents

Purchasers of this book can download
and print an enlarged version of the Appendix
at *www.guilford.com/jurist-forms*
for personal use or use with individual
clients (see copyright page for details).

Introduction

Not less than knowing, doubting pleases me.
—DANTE, *The Inferno*[1]

We often do not know what we feel. This simple but striking point has been taken for granted in the proliferating literature on emotions. Of course, this does not mean we are always ignorant of our feelings or that we cannot move in the direction of knowing and using our emotions effectively. It only suggests that the meaning(s) of our emotions elude even our best effort to understand them. Moreover, there is no ready assurance that our assessments are accurate or that we are not retroactively inventing reasons to justify our emotions (Haidt, 2001; Kurzban & Aktipis, 2007). Acknowledging that we do not fully know what we feel is crucial, as it encourages caution and humility in the way we construe our potential for "emotional intelligence" or "emotion regulation." The experience of not knowing our feelings is an everyday part of our lives, and certainly not just true for the subset of humanity who happen to seek out psychotherapy.

As I discuss in Chapter 1, I have introduced the term "aporetic emotions" to capture the experience of emotions dwelling within us as obscure, mystifying, or confusing mental states (Jurist, 2005). The Socratic ring is intentional, as I submit it is better to know that we do not know than to think we know (and be wrong) or to know in a facile way.

---

[1]This famous line is in the sixth circle of hell, when Dante responds to Virgil concerning the sins of incontinence. The passage is cited in Manguel (2015), who also cites Montaigne's use of it.

1

When it comes to emotions, it is difficult to escape from the land between ignorance and knowledge.[2] Nevertheless, my study will focus on the challenge of engaging with aporetic emotions and potentially moving beyond them by identifying, modulating, and expressing emotions.

My full answer as to how it might be possible to transcend aporetic emotions is through mentalizing them. Mentalization, a concept of growing importance in philosophy and in many subdisciplines in psychology, denotes that the mind interprets reality and utilizes skills that produce self-understanding and understanding others. Derived from diverse sources that I explicate in Chapter 4, mentalization has been taken up in psychoanalysis as a new way to capture the importance of the relationship or therapeutic alliance. Therapists mentalize about their patients' mental states and invite patients to mentalize about their own mental states and about others' (including their therapists'). As I will argue, mentalizing represents a unique gloss on therapeutic action and the goals of psychotherapy.

Success in psychotherapy depends on patients' improvement as mentalizers. Indeed, all psychotherapy boils down to being a project of two minds engaging each other and trying to make sense together. Mentalization is based on a range of skills that can be cultivated in therapy; it fosters an abiding way to negotiate life and relationships, and where suffering exists, to cope with it optimally. Mentalization alters the traditional goal of psychotherapy away from either self-knowledge or behavioral change. In place of these, the ideal is for patients to work on communication, valuing the input from others and being vulnerable in revealing themselves. Epistemic trust, the capacity for infants to rely on learning from caregivers, and epistemic vigilance, the capacity for young children to discern who to trust, are necessary in order for communication to emerge that is based on valuing truthfulness. Mentalizing is akin to open-mindedness, wherein we sustain an active, fallible investment in reevaluation of self and others, past and present.

Mentalized affectivity is the specific aspect of mentalizing that is most germane to psychotherapy. It bears some kinship to "emotion regulation," but emphasizes that emotions are mediated through the prism of autobiographical memory (AM) (Fonagy, Gergely, Jurist, &

---

[2]Indeed, this is debatably true for all spheres of learning. Firestein (2012) and Holmes (2015) mount compelling arguments that even in science, knowledge is less certain than it often appears, and they stress that doubt and ambiguity should be embraced and valued, rather than dismissed. Harari (2015) urges us to recall that modern science begins with admitting ignorance and the awareness of "we do not know" (p. 250), which thrived under the marriage of science and empire as the discovery of unknown continents was pursued, and even more so under the economic incentives of capitalism.

Target, 2002; Jurist, 2005, 2008, 2010, 2014). The source of mentalized affectivity lies in curiosity, the desire to understand how one's past and identity inform one's emotional experience, and its fruition is manifest in the love of truth, or truthfulness, the desire to face oneself and others as honestly as possible. In pushing us to make sense of our current emotional experience in light of AM, mentalized affectivity provides a critical perspective by which we can observe, question, and refashion ourselves, insofar as that is possible to do.[3]

Although my own therapeutic approach is psychodynamic, what I propose about working with emotions will be relevant to all therapists, regardless of orientation. Ultimately, my approach will be to introduce ways to help patients access and reflect on emotions, tools that can be combined with a wide range of techniques. In order to grasp the complexity of emotional experience, it will be helpful to look beyond research studies and include examples that come from diverse sources such as clinical vignettes and autobiographical writing. The clinical vignettes I present in this book are snapshots, or better yet, "snapchats," brief, instantaneous, revealing moments with patients. This style will allow us to glimpse lived emotional experience without compromising ethical standards around confidentiality. Details about the patients have been altered to protect their identities.

The memoirs that I cite are wide-ranging: a comedian in Chapter 1 (Sarah Silverman), a poet in Chapter 2 (Tracy K. Smith), a filmmaker in Chapter 3 (Ingmar Bergman), and a neurologist/writer in Chapter 5 (Oliver Sacks). Autobiographical memoirs are a burgeoning field of literature; indeed, I have begun writing this Introduction on the same day that the Book Review section of the *New York Times* has commenced a regular feature by Meghan Daum, called "Egos." Autobiographical narratives provide a measure of our culture at a particular juncture in time, and transcend merely being a record of private life. To some extent, autobiographical narratives might be considered as a kind of therapeutic endeavor, given the positive benefits of putting thoughts into words (Pennebaker, 1997).

My choice of memoirs, out of the many types of illustration that might have been selected, is based on their creative insight into lived

---

[3] Reber's (2016) notion of "critical feeling" seems closely related to my idea of mentalized affectivity: "the reflective use of feelings that is focused on guiding attention, evaluating information, and guiding action according to the values we like to implement" (p. 60). Reber defends the idea of strategizing with our emotions mainly from a social psychology rather than a clinical perspective. Although he does mention how critical feeling might be incorporated into psychotherapy, he is especially interested in its wide application to education, business and politics, the arts, and religion.

emotional experience. They are exemplary in that they provide rich, reflective data about emotions, both personally and culturally. Memoirs depict emotions actually and contextually. For the record, I do not assume the clinical vignettes I cite necessarily reflect psychopathology; nor that autobiographical narratives are immune from psychological difficulties. It is an atypical but deliberate choice to mix clinical and nonclinical material, as both serve to supplement the current state of scientific research on emotions. Emotions are vexing enough to require any and all means of study.

The book has two parts. Part I has three chapters aimed at equipping therapists to help people experience and utilize their emotions (and to consider specific problems with emotions). Chapter 1 focuses on identifying emotions. I argue that identifying emotions is not as straightforward as it might seem; I discuss the idea mentioned above, of "aporetic emotions," and I elaborate on problems in identifying emotions in relation to research about alexithymia. I provide various examples: patients who can identify some emotions but not others; patients who talk around emotions; and patients who tend to omit them. I focus on Sarah Silverman's history and especially her experience of the emotion of fear and how she transformed it through performing onstage, although she remains burdened by its presence.

Chapter 2 focuses on modulating emotions. Here I introduce recent work on emotion regulation, specifically the process model, which emphasizes cognitive reappraisal, and also the mindfulness model, which serves as a critique of the process model in encouraging acceptance rather than transformation of emotions. I discuss the importance of emotion regulation in development, especially in relation to the self, and also research on how emotion dysregulation underlies many kinds of psychopathology. I discuss several measures of emotion regulation. A number of examples offered in this chapter demonstrate the struggle to regulate emotions upwardly and downwardly. Notably, my examples point to the relational quality of regulation: that we rely on others in order to self-regulate. I use Tracy K. Smith's memoir, which is a meditation on her mourning for her mother who died when Smith was quite young (22 years old). I also raise limits, questions, and reservations about emotion regulation as a concept.

Chapter 3 focuses on expressing emotions. I make a distinction between the inward and outward expression of emotions, and I consider examples of effective and not so effective communication. I discuss the heterogeneity of expressing emotions and introduce some measures of the expression of emotions. I also emphasize how culture influences the trajectory of expression. Ingmar Bergman's autobiographical memoir documents his struggle to express his emotions, especially to others, in spite of his brilliant and subtle depiction of emotions in his films.

There is a sequential logic throughout the first three chapters in the sense that it helps to express emotions well if one modulates emotions, and it helps to modulate emotions if one identifies them. The movement from identifying to modulating to expressing requires an increase in the exercise of agency: identifying represents the inception of agency, modulating the actualization of agency, and expressing the realization of agency. Yet, there are tricky questions about how identifying, modulating, and expressing emotions blend into each other, and whether they are dialectically and intrinsically related insofar as they all have to do with selves seeking to find meaning in emotions. The Coda at the end of Part I includes reflection on the relation among the categories of identifying, modulating, and expressing emotions. I compare the three autobiographical memoirs that are discussed in terms of the extent to which one's history and identity account for one's experience of emotions.

Part II comprises four chapters that delve into the experience of mentalizing emotions. Chapter 4 explores the concept of mentalization, where it comes from, and how it illuminates our understanding of emotion, culminating with "mentalized affectivity," the term I have introduced to the literature. I briefly discuss the Mentalized Affectivity Scale (MAS), which my research team has created (see the Appendix for the measure itself and scoring instructions). In this chapter, I illustrate how Peter Fonagy and colleagues have articulated the concept of mentalization in an original way by integrating diverse strands from the cognitive sciences and French psychoanalysis. I describe current measures of reflective function, the operationalized concept of mentalization. I also speculate about aspects of mentalization that are in need of clarification and refinement. This chapter is theoretical and serves as an introduction to mentalization theory.

Chapter 5 develops the concept of mentalized affectivity in more detail and incorporates recent research on AM along with clinical illustrations. I review literature on the relation among AM, narrative, and self, and I compare my understanding and measure of mentalized affectivity to related ones in the field. I introduce clinical vignettes of low, medium, and high mentalizers. I turn to examine Oliver Sacks's two autobiographies, which are quite different in tone, and I reflect on the impact of his nearly 50 years working with the same psychoanalyst. Sacks wrote a number of short autobiographical pieces in the *New York Times*, a record of his final thoughts, which together with his two autobiographical works provide a superb illustration of mentalized affectivity.

Chapter 6 focuses on mentalized affectivity as therapeutic action. The term "therapeutic action" signifies the ideal that psychotherapy can inspire ongoing change, aspiring to a higher goal beyond symptom relief. Mentalized affectivity helps us to realize the ultimate goal of psychotherapy: communication. The kind of communication that mentalized affectivity supports is based on the love of truth or truthfulness, the desire to tell and hear the truth, the value of pursuing and claiming truth, however elusive it might be. In this chapter, I focus on the dynamics of self and other between the patient and therapist, utilizing the idea of epistemic circumspection, and I end by reflecting on psychotherapy as a social institution, based on the communication paradigm.

In Chapter 7, I locate mentalized affectivity in relation to other psychoanalytic ideas and theories—like the Bionian and post-Bionian appreciation of the rudimentary communication of emotions (or proto-emotions, which resemble aporetic emotions), and the emphasis on collaboration, mutual mentalizing, and the specific positionalities of the therapist and patient in relational psychoanalysis. I suggest that mentalized affectivity needs to integrate these ideas, and at the same time, that the construct has the potential to lead contemporary psychoanalytic theory forward. Mentalized affectivity affirms the value of communication, and, as I argue, communication relies upon truthfulness. The communication paradigm represents a shift away from attachment in mentalization theory, given that attachment is a shared function between humans and animals. The relationship enables truthfulness to thrive; so, it matters, but not exclusively.

The Conclusion spells out the larger implications of my study in terms of overcoming the worsening disconnect between the scientific and literary cultures. I examine the specific case of clinical psychology as a field and reflect on current trends in the mental health profession. I worry about the mentality of science and nothing but science, and argue in favor of more creative efforts to include both science and literature, as I have tried to do throughout this study.

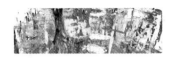 **PART I**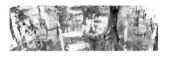

IDENTIFYING, MODULATING, AND EXPRESSING EMOTIONS

Emotions are not detached theoretical states; they address a practical concern from a personal and interested perspective.
—AARON BEN-ZE'EV, "The Logic of Emotions" (2003)

 **CHAPTER 1**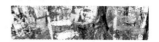

Identifying Emotions

Knowing a feeling requires a knower subject.
—ANTONIO R. DAMASIO, *The Feeling of What Happens* (1999)

Although we sometimes know what we feel with clarity, it is hardly uncommon for us to be unsure, mystified, or even conflicted. It can be an indication of psychopathology not to know what we feel, but that certainly does not have to be the case. Our understanding of such phenomena is not well developed, and correspondingly our language for describing it is rather limited. The term "alexithymia" overlaps with what I am getting at, as I discuss in more detail later in this chapter. However, alexithymia tends to imply a general impairment in being able to know one's feelings, whereas what I have in mind can be situational as well as occasional. The fact that we do not always know what we feel is important, as it is vastly underestimated in contemporary accounts of emotion. For example, the basic emotions theory, which has become the dominant (but not unchallenged) approach in the study of emotions, supposes that emotions have a quick onset, brief duration, and rely on automatic appraisal (Ekman & Davidson, 1994). If we are interested in casting a wider net and, in particular, understanding how emotions are lived, rather than how they have been studied, we need to pay close attention to states of not being sure of what one is feeling.

APORETIC EMOTIONS

Alexithymia is a useful and promising personality trait that correlates with diagnoses, but it should be supplemented by a term that denotes confusion or uncertainty, without the connotation of lacking the ability to know one's feelings. A good way to characterize what I am aiming to describe is the term "aporetic emotions," that is, emotions that are vague and lack sharp specificity. Aporetic emotions manifest themselves when we know we feel something but we are not sure what it is, and the effort to fathom those feelings seems directionless or blocked. The introduction of this term is helpful, too, in reminding us that we often feel a partial, confusing mixture of the so-called basic emotions, not simply one of them. The term "aporetic" literally means "*a* = not" and "*poria* = crossable," taken from the inconclusive results of Socratic dialogue. It is a term associated with questioning and skepticism, but it is meant to connote the *difficulty* of acquiring knowledge, not necessarily its impossibility.

Patients come to therapy all the time knowing that they feel something but not being sure what it is. Partners turn to their significant others regularly in the same state. The introduction of this term marks my concern that there are obstacles to emotional intelligence and emotion regulation that ought to be recognized. Let us consider an example from Stephen Grosz's *The Examined Life* (2013). The patient, Matt, a young man (21 years old) who had been adopted at 2 years old, had gotten in trouble for pointing an unloaded starter pistol at a police officer and subsequently acting out in various ways. Grosz notices his own lack of engagement with Matt and attributes it to the "sort of gap between what a person says and what he makes you feel," which he adds is "not uncommon" (p. 24). Grosz connects his reaction to Matt's estranged relation to his own emotions:

> I began to realize that Matt did not register his own emotions. In the course of our two-hour conversation, he seemed either to pick up and employ my descriptions of his feelings or to infer his emotions from the behavior of others. For example, he said he didn't know why he had pointed the gun at the police officer. I suggested he might have been angry. "Yeah, I was angry," Matt replied. "What did you feel when you were angry?" I asked. "You know, the police, they were very angry with me. My parents were very angry with me. Everyone was very angry with me," he replied. "But what did you feel?" I asked. "They were all shouting at me," he told me. (pp. 25–26)

Not only does Matt confuse the way others (the police, his parents) feel with how he feels, but he obscures his motivation for the action with the reaction others had to what he did. Grosz sees Matt as an extreme case, and with more information, we might be inclined to see him as alexithymic. Yet, Grosz chooses to conclude his mini–case discussion by emphasizing a point that I agree with: "There is a bit of Matt in each of us" (p. 27).

There are a few other descriptions I have encountered that are relevant to aporetic emotions. The first example comes from popular psychology, a recent headline and story by Webber (2016) on "odd emotions," which defy labels and do not fit into any neat categories. The second example comes from the Italian post-Bionian psychoanalyst Antonino Ferro (2011), who introduces the notion of "proto-emotions," emotions that make themselves felt but are not formed. The idea here is that they are not formed because it would be too threatening to do so. As I discuss in more detail in Chapter 6, Ferro understands proto-emotions as having content that a person is not able to recognize. While it is important to appreciate that it can be more ego-syntonic not to experience emotions, in my view, not all aporetic emotions are proto-emotions; the former is a larger category of which the latter is a part.

My understanding of aporetic emotions corresponds to the subjective aspect of what Damasio (2010) has termed "primordial feelings" in his neuroscientific account of the evolution of the self. Primordial emotions occur through the brain monitoring the state of the body; they precede other more specific emotions and tend to have a valence of pleasure or pain. Following Panksepp (1998), Damasio sees the construction of the self (or proto-self) as generating primordial feelings, which come from brain-stem nuclei. Damasio's main claim is that all normal mental states include some form of feeling; he is less interested in the vague uncertainty that I have ascribed to (and that I believe defines) aporetic emotions. In a previous book, *The Feeling of What Happens* (1999), Damasio invokes Daniel Stern's (1985) developmental notion of "vitality affects" in connection to primordial emotions (p. 287). At the heart of Damasio's (2010) argument, though, is an evolutionary hypothesis, which suggests that feelings can be mixed states, produced from different brain sites (p. 112). Although this view is speculative, it seems appealing to understand aporetic emotions as linked to the evolution of the brain.

Aporetic emotions can be fleeting and come in and out of focus. Happily, it is sometimes possible to get better at recognizing what one feels, and to have success experiencing and managing emotions. Making such progress, in my experience, requires developing curiosity about emotions. With every patient I encounter, I ask myself whether the person seems curious about his or her emotions. If a patient seems not to be curious about emotions, I accept that the going will be slow and adjust the pace accordingly. But how can one promote curiosity about emotions where there is none?

I have succeeded in inspiring patients to be curious about emotions, to appreciate what is at stake in pursuing this effort, rather than ignoring it. Of course, I have also failed, and can distinguish between absolute failures, where there simply is no progress, and cases where the patient makes a concession to acknowledge that identifying emotions is necessary in order to function better in life. It is possible, I believe, to be invested in identifying emotions prior to having much curiosity about them.

In some unusual cases, there is not only a lack of curiosity about emotions, but something more perverse, where there is a kind of automatic rejection of emotions. This can shade into the bizarre phenomenon in which emotions, when felt, are reflexively expulsed. It is very sad to encounter a person who finds his or her own emotions to be toxic, since this would have to limit the capacity to enjoy life and give and take pleasure from others. Most people have some attachment to their own emotions and are receptive to the challenge of identifying, modulating, and expressing them. In this chapter, I look closely at vicissitudes and complexities around the task of identifying emotions.

FEAR AND PERFORMANCE: SARAH SILVERMAN

Identifying emotions is not as straightforward as it might seem at first glance. As I have suggested, it is a mistake to assume that whenever we feel something, we know what it is. Often, an emotion is experienced as found—like walking down a street at night and suddenly experiencing a sense of fear wash over you. Other times, identifying emotions can entail more of a search—like when a patient heard about a promotion that would require more time away from his family, resulting in oscillation among quite different emotions (from elation at being rewarded to worry about not being around the daily life of his family). Finally, identifying emotions can involve an active negotiation of a conflict—as when a patient discussed her reaction to hearing about the death of the mother of an ex-boyfriend (from whom she had parted unhappily).

When one thinks about identifying emotions, it will usually be about one's own emotions, but it can also be about others' emotions. There has not been much attention in the literature to identifying emotions that belong to others, especially not having to do with early life development. Clearly, this phenomenon is too important to ignore, as being able to identify the emotions of others must have an impact on intimate relationships and social life. We do not really know, for example, whether it is possible to be adept at identifying one's own emotions but inept at identifying the emotions of others (or vice versa). It is tempting, for example, to speculate about how identifying one's own or others' emotions links to psychopathology: that borderline personalities focus on the emotions of others at the expense of their own, and narcissists focus on their own emotions at the expense of others (Diamond, Yeomans, & Stern, 2018). We cannot simply assume that if one cares about emotions, one is able to identify them within oneself or with others. Identifying emotions as internal states might require different skills compared to identifying emotions by relying on the data revealed through facial expressions.

How much time and effort one needs to put into identifying emotions varies. It seems possible and even, on occasion, desirable to act on an emotion without first identifying it: Oh, my God, that's not a dog, it's a mountain lion! Moreover, it is impossible to escape the issue of context—in the examples mentioned above, it matters whether the fearful person had ever been mugged, whether the patient who was promoted has been happy in his career choice, and what the relationship between the patient and her ex's mother had been like. Indeed, it seems almost artificial to imagine that we would be invested in identifying emotions with no valence about how one feels about being in that emotional state.

Another way to make this point is to stress that we all have feelings about our feelings. Most of us like to feel joy and would prefer not to feel afraid; other emotions are trickier to make generalizations about. For example, it is always fascinating how differently people react to being angry: some find anger to be like a hot potato, that once it is apparent, it needs to be disposed of, versus others for whom anger is ego-syntonic and who are happy to become angry at the least provocation.

The fact that we have feelings about our feelings sometimes manifests itself as one emotion standing in place of another. In other words, emotions can perform the work that psychoanalysts have attributed to defenses—displacing uncomfortable emotions away from awareness. Greenberg's (2015) emotion-focused therapy offers excellent examples of how secondary emotions are utilized to conceal primary emotions. For example, how sadness, the primary emotion, can be masked by and underlie anger, the secondary emotion (p. 226). According to Greenberg, we can distinguish between so-called primary emotions, which concern a core feeling about the self and, when identified, are experienced like arriving at a destination, and so-called secondary emotions, which serve to block access to primary feelings. I am not convinced that the emotions behind emotions can be explicated in terms of the neat distinction between primary and secondary, but the emotion-focused therapy approach helps us to appreciate the complexity of identifying emotions.

The etymology of the word "identify" is telling, as it includes not just naming, but seeing oneself as alike to something. Moreover, it is worth keeping in mind that the etymology of "identify" is related to "identity." In other words, in identifying emotions, we are bringing our identity with us. Identifying is spurred by curiosity, and so identifying does not end with a name, but can continue as a form of exploration.

Let us consider an example of identifying emotions from an autobiography. Comedian Sarah Silverman's memoir is titled *The Bedwetter* (2010) and documents, as advertised, her enuresis; it is the kind of autobiographical writing where the author dwells on her most private feelings. Silverman relates a painful history (the first chapter is titled "Cursed from the Start"), which includes the death of a sibling (a crib accident prior to her birth), her parents' divorce (which emerges out of sequence and is not discussed at all), and the suicide of her therapist (another therapist in the practice blurts out that he hung himself as she awaits her appointment). Silverman explains that she heard about the death of her brother as a kind of campfire ghost story told by her older sister. It is revealing that she did not hear this from her parents, and it is unclear if her parents learned that she knew or spoke with her about this tragic event. In any case, Silverman movingly observes that "It lived in the front of my mind for a long time after" (p. 15). Toward the end of the memoir, Silverman tells us that her parents divorced when she was 7 years old (p. 222), although an allusion to this had been introduced in connection to her father's understanding of her enuresis and need to see a therapist. The story of arriving for an appointment only to be told that her therapist had hung himself is awful, and Silverman understandably muses whether there might have been a more professional way for the other therapist to handle the situation.

Despite depicting these dramatic events, Silverman's memoir is easy to read, the bathos mixed with an edge of not taking herself too seriously. She is determined to entertain us throughout. Silverman is adept at presenting herself as bored by the project, while occasionally displaying vulnerability and being self-revealing. She uses different voices to play with the reader. For example, Silverman begins the book with a Foreword, which contrary to her editor's recommendation, she insists on writing herself, establishing a meta-level space to observe herself. The book also contains a Midword, which allows Silverman to refer to the Foreword as an "autoforeword," and to the self-mocking association of writing a book and masturbating. The book concludes with a blasphemous Afterword, allegedly written by God, that forecasts Silverman's future life.

Silverman's enuresis is a central theme in the memoir, as the full title suggests: *The Bedwetter: Stories of Courage, Redemption, and Pee.* It is clinically noteworthy that this problem was transgenerational: both her father and grandfather had suffered from it (p. 37). Silverman's enuresis is linked to anxiety and causes her to have repeated experiences of humiliation, ultimately contributing to becoming depressed as an adolescent for 3 years. Silverman informs us that she missed 3 straight months of ninth grade because of being "paralyzed with fear" (p. 34). She identifies the emotion of fear but construes it as part of a larger context of growing up feeling confused, alone, and depressed. Silverman moves on to elaborate on her early life trauma as a gift, though, as her paralyzing fear yielded to fearlessness and natural comfort performing in front of others (p. 74). It turns out that bedwetting is retrospectively interpreted as a source of triumphant success as well as an image of amusing self-deprecation. Let us take note of how this real-life example of identifying the emotion of fear is set against the background context of depression and ultimately provides the opportunity for self-overcoming. The basic emotion in and of itself is embedded in her life experience. Revealingly, Silverman's point is not that she felt and then overcame fear. As she reflects:

> The truth is, from that time up to now, *inside,* I haven't changed. My outer shell may mutate, I may come to embrace the things that scare and upset me, but it all comes from the same *place.* At some point, I figured that it would be far more effective and far funnier to embrace the ugliest, most terrifying things in the world—the Holocaust, racism, rape, et cetera. But for the sake of comedy, and the comedian's personal sanity, this requires a certain emotional distance. . . . But adopting a persona at once ignorant and arrogant allowed me to say what I didn't mean, even preach the opposite of what I believed. For me, it was a funny way to be sincere. And like the jokes in a roast, the hope is that the genuine sentiment—maybe even a *goodness* underneath the joke (however brutal) transcends. (pp. 156–157; original emphasis)[1]

This revealing self-reflection demonstrates how troublesome emotions, once identified, do not disappear, although they can be used in such a way that they do not plague us, and, in fact, can be mobilized in new directions of freeing oneself and connecting with others. Silverman's primary emotion of fear does not dissipate; rather, its dangerous power is kept at bay in creative new ways. Making sense of emotions

---

[1] In this same passage, Silverman draws an interesting parallel between the comedian and the shrink, stressing the need for the capacity for emotional distance: "It really takes someone strong, someone, I dare say, with a big fat wall up—to work in a pool of heartbreak all day and not want to fucking kill yourself" (pp. 156–157). I take this as a salutary plea to therapists to love our defenses and not to ignore our own needs in our determination to be empathic with and toward patients. Silverman invoked the wisdom of her own therapist in her comments at the Democratic National Convention in Philadelphia in July 2016. Recently, she has participated in a video series that aims to destigmatize therapy (see Yandoli, 2017).

that one has identified shades into a further activity, that is, modulating emotions, which I focus on in the next chapter.

Silverman uses the memoir to describe and advocate a spirit of moderation with her favorite motto, "make it a treat," which she explains as a strenuous effort to resist excess. Interestingly, too, at the 2016 Democratic convention, Silverman made a strong, reasonable pitch to supporters of Bernie Sanders to embrace Hillary Clinton, which garnered considerable attention. She appeared with the former comedian and now former senator Al Franken, who figures in the memoir in that Silverman and he worked together as writers at *Saturday Night Live*. Ironically enough, Franken had been the object of a strange act of impulsivity described in the book, where Silverman attempted to put a pencil through his curly hair but struck him in the forehead. In accounting for her action, Silverman describes her emotions as aporetic: "I don't think I thought with actual words. It's weird now to try to articulate it that way. However, the mind works when it's not forming sentences—with pictures maybe? I guess, yes . . . " (p. 111). Although pictorial images might themselves have clarity, there is still a gap implied here between what she feels and what she can put into words.

The emotion of fear is prominent in Silverman's saga—not only is she able to identify it, but she demonstrates that we *can do* things with emotions. So, identifying emotions is not just a matter of providing them with a name or label. Identifying emotions can mean different things for different people in different contexts; however, it does presume a certain curiosity about emotions. Fear, the emotion that plagued Silverman while she was growing up, is utilized as motivation for her to become a successful performer.

PROBLEMS IN IDENTIFYING EMOTIONS

In the context of psychotherapy, it is endlessly interesting to see how patients choose to divulge their emotions. Patients, by definition, come because they are suffering from something, and they deserve credit for making the choice to seek help. It should go without saying, too, that just because someone is *not* in psychotherapy, it does not necessarily mean that that person might not need or benefit from help.

When it comes to emotions, some patients identify emotions explicitly, using the appropriate emotion word in a way that makes sense. For example, characterizing a minor "dis" from a friend in terms of annoyance, rather than anger or rage. Patients can also use emotion words in idiosyncratic or self-serving ways—like a patient who refers to himself as a little anxious in the context of describing an argument with his wife where there had been a threat of violence. It is often productive to flesh this out with some patients, who might be tempted to engage in the equivalent of copping to a lesser crime, while, in fact, minimizing or disowning their real feelings. However, patients can also be quite unaware of how their use of emotion words departs from customary usage.

So, patients can name the emotion (appropriately or not), or they can avoid this (defensively or because they are unaware of what they are feeling). Another variation occurs with patients who have a way of talking around the emotion without being explicit about it. I recall one patient who had no trouble identifying specific emotions but was more inclined to tell me about what he thought he should feel, rather than what he actually felt. He would use the introductory phrase "I was a little upset . . . " in an overly generalized way, not marking degrees and minimizing his real, more complicated feelings. During our work, we explored this, and he began to realize that he feared exposing his feelings because he assumed he would be compelled to act on them. It was not easy for him to divulge his actual feelings, as he worried, too, that I would try to dissuade him from living up to his ideals.

It is important to consider whether patients are able to appreciate how emotions can be combined, and not just discern single emotions. For example, a patient became tearful in response to a comment from me about how she was working hard in therapy. She realized that my words had touched her and made her feel good but served to remind her that her mother never said things like this and she always wished that she had done so.

It is worth pausing to wonder why it is important to identify feelings. Although it is fair to assume that it is beneficial to know one's feelings, let us consider this with a view toward a better understanding of mental health. In some ways, it has to be an advantage for the sake of survival to be able to identify one's feelings. In addition, identifying one's feelings is conducive to self-knowledge: knowing what one feels is a part of knowing one's self. It is debatable whether identifying feelings ought to contribute to happiness. Preliminary results from my research suggest that while subjects readily value identifying emotions, it is not strongly linked to life satisfaction (Greenberg, Kolasi, Hegsted, Berkowitz, & Jurist, 2017).

From one perspective, identifying feelings ought to lead us in the direction of fathoming unhappiness. From another perspective, though, identifying feelings might be linked to experiencing a wide palette of emotions, across the domains of positive and negative affect. As Shedler (2010) has argued, the aim of psychotherapy should not be restricted to decreasing symptoms, but to seeking psychological health, which includes a full exploration of affects. This would mean treatment would entail helping patients not to identify some feelings at the expense of others, but to be open to experiencing an ample range of affects.

In my view, identifying emotions is crucial because it facilitates communication. Knowing what one feels enables a person to share (or not) that information with others. Sharing information helps to build and sustain trust in relationships. Insofar as one has such relationships, identifying emotions can foster improved specificity and detail. Insofar as one does not have such relationships, psychotherapy can be understood as providing a practice space in which the patient can experiment with being understood and cultivating a better understanding of one's own mental states. As Fonagy and Allison (2014) argue, therapy offers the opportunity for patients with severe personality disorders to rekindle epistemic trust where it has been lost. For other patients, epistemic trust can enlarge and actualize self-understanding. I discuss this in more detail in Chapters 4 and 6.

ALEXITHYMIA AND CULTURE

Persistent difficulties in being able to identify emotions portend larger problems and an increased likelihood of psychopathology. In this section, I amplify how difficulty in identifying emotions can be linked to general and specific forms of psychopathology. Yet, keep in mind that all of us can improve our ability to identify emotions.

The concept that is most relevant to problems in identifying emotions, as previously noted, is alexithymia. Alexithymia denotes deficits in subjective awareness and cognitive processing of emotions, and it is closely linked to psychosomatics in that emotions that cannot be tolerated mentally are construed in terms of bodily states. Taylor, Bagby, and Parker (1997) describe the salient features of alexithymia as "(i) difficulty identifying feelings and distinguishing between feelings and the bodily sensations of emotional arousal; (ii) difficulty describing feelings to other people; (iii) constricted imaginal processes, as evidenced by a paucity of fantasies; and (iv) a stimulus-bound, externally orientated cognitive style" (p. 29).

A virtue of the construct of alexithymia is that it has been operationalized and measured empirically. The Toronto Alexithymia Scale (TAS-20) describes the construct as referring to people "who have trouble identifying and describing emotions and who tend to minimize emotional experience and focus attention externally" (Bagby, Parker, & Taylor, 1994). The TAS-20 has three factors: (1) difficulty identifying feelings; (2) difficulty describing feelings, and (3) externally-oriented thinking (TAS-20). The scale has demonstrated good internal consistency (.81) and test–retest reliability (.77), and has been found stable and replicable across both clinical and nonclinical populations. A more recent scale, the Toronto Structured Interview for Alexithymia (TSIA), was created in 2006 to address the fact that the TAS-20 relies on self-report, which might be confounding for the population in question; according to the authors, the TSIA seems to correlate well with the TAS-20 (Taylor & Bagby, 2013).

As a construct, alexithymia captures a phenomenon that had not been previously been described or appreciated. It is a broader construct than identifying emotions: people with alexithymia have problems over and beyond identifying emotions. Alexithymia has been linked to a number of different kinds of psychopathology: autism spectrum disorders, schizophrenia, addictions, eating disorders, personality disorders, and posttraumatic stress disorder (PTSD). Evidence for these links varies; for example, personality disorders have been linked to externally oriented thinking, but not to identifying feelings (De Panfilis, Ossala, Tonna, Catania, & Marchesi, 2015). Difficulty in identifying feelings has been linked to somatization independent of somatic diseases, anxiety, and depression (Mattila et al., 2008; Taylor & Bagby, 2013).

Alexithymia is conceived as a personality trait that maps onto various psychopathologies. However, as Taylor and Bagby (2013) have argued, its legacy extends back to psychoanalysis and psychosomatics. One important source, which I elaborate on in Chapter 4, lies in the "dementalizing" that Pierre Marty detected in patients who rely on "pensée opératoire," a kind of concrete thinking devoid of fantasy or recalled dreams, and in which little symbolic activity takes place. Bouchard and Lecours (2008) explicate operative thinking in terms of tangential associations, words that reduplicate action, stereotyped expressions, clichés, and conformism, thoughts and memories that are not related in a coherent framework, not using context to create meaning, and an empty presence (or "white relationship") that lacks reference to an inner, live object or self (pp. 110–111). Marty (Marty & M'Uzan, 1963) suggests that people who fit this description live as if everything happens or is imposed on them (p. 348). Somatizing occurs in the face of failing to mentalize, where what happens in the mind is read as if it is happening in the body. In other words, as Gubb (2013) avows, "The mind cannot express itself as a mind because it is all body" (p. 117).

Although the origins of the term "alexithymia" go back to the 1950s, it was only in the 1970s and 1980s that an appreciation arose for how widespread a phenomenon this was. The work of McDougall (1989) and Krystal (1988) suggests that trauma might be the source of alexithymia. The correlation between alexithymia and trauma has been supported in recent research (Kano & Fukudo, 2013), specifically that insecure attachment fosters problems with experiencing emotions. Another study linked alexithymia to a dismissing, devaluing style of attachment and negatively to a style of secure attachment (Scheidt et al., 1999). It seems reasonable to suppose that people who have avoidant attachment histories and who tend toward being schizoid would especially struggle to be able to identify emotions. However, identifying emotions, as I have repeatedly emphasized, can be at issue for anyone.

The link between alexithymia and attachment inspires us to wonder about the origins of alexithymia as well as how we might think about treating it. In considering a developmental perspective, though, I do not mean to discount other perspectives, such as a neurobiological one. For example, it has been demonstrated that alexithymics have less activation in brain areas associated with emotional awareness in viewing facial expressions (Kano & Fukida, 2013). So, it is a combination of factors that will impact one's ability to identify emotions.

In addition to a developmental and neurobiological perspective, a cultural perspective is worth considering. The challenge of identifying emotions cannot be divorced from the fact that emotions are part of larger meaning systems. This is consistent with the views of those, like Tomkins (1995), who have drawn attention to emotions as packaged in scripts that tell us what they mean. Yet, there is a deeper sense of how culture influences emotions, which many scholars have argued, wherein the same emotion can mean very different things in the logic of cultures (Markus & Kitiyama, 1991; Russell, 1991; Shweder, 1994). Indeed, there is a large and growing literature on cross-cultural aspects of emotions, which ought to make us sensitive to the fact that as clinicians, we are interested in what the patient means by naming an emotion. Some of my clinical examples will give expression to this point.

We can also view alexithymia from a postmodern perspective. People negotiate among past, current, and evolving cultural beliefs, and, in particular, there is less of a consensus about emotions than in the past. All of us—not just suffering patients—face the task of figuring out to what extent culturally prescribed practices fit our personal beliefs. Therapy is often sought out precisely as the realm in which one can freely articulate and confront these issues. Giddens (1992) maintains that a transformation has occurred in our understanding of sexuality and intimacy, where the restrictions of the past become subject to the democratizing process of free choice and self-determination, which applies to our emotions as well. Some recent examples of our postmodern dilemma are manifest in popular culture: David Brooks's book *The Road to Character* (2015) and Disney's big hit *Inside Out* ostensibly point to finding hopeful, palatable solutions but ultimately document and reflect the extent to which virtues and emotions, however important, lack consensus in our current cultural self-understanding. In short, identifying emotions runs up against valuing emotions.

IDENTIFYING VIGNETTES

Let us now begin to turn our attention to the clinical realm and translate what I have been suggesting into practice. Some patients come to therapy being fairly comfortable and adept at identifying emotions. For those patients who do come to therapy having difficulty with identifying emotions, it's imperative that therapists focus on this and devise ways to improve their ability.

Along with others, Krystal (1988) has argued that psychoeducation is necessary to help patients who are not able to identify emotions. Krystal also maintains that treatment with such patients needs to be supportive rather than interpretive, aimed at helping them tolerate their experience. I would agree to a certain extent, especially with the emphasis on the therapist's potential need to accept going slower and refrain from making assumptions that might be beyond where the patient is. However, I am uneasy with the supposition that the therapist can tell a patient what it means to feel a specific emotion. I submit we're more likely to succeed if we enlist the patient in a process of actively considering this for him- or herself. This follows from what I have said about the cultural and postmodernist aspects of emotions. Alexander's (1953) old-school wisdom advocating the emotionally corrective experience unwittingly portrays the analyst as (omnipotently) able to tell the patient what he or she feels. My reservation on this point helps to differentiate my perspective from Greenberg's emotion-focused therapy, which relies on coaches who are didactic and instruct their clients about what they are feeling.

I would characterize my approach to helping patients identify emotions in terms of mentalization, which will be discussed in Chapter 4 and thereafter in Part II. Identifying emotions entails a process in which the therapist joins the patient in naming, understanding, and tolerating his or her feelings. There is room still for the analyst to say how he or she sees things, but it is never ideal for a clinician to assume the posture of having a superior relation to reality. Moreover, unless a therapist knows a patient well, he or she ought to be cautious about ascribing feelings to the patient. Taylor and Bagby (2013) have offered an argument with which I concur: that treating alexithymic patients means helping them to mentalize their emotions. A series of questions can be formulated to support inquiry about what the patient is feeling: Why does the patient think it is difficult for him or her to identify an emotional state? Does the patient name some emotions and not name others? Does the patient explain what he or she means by referring to an emotion? Is the meaning, insofar as it is specified, appropriate or idiosyncratic? Although I am mentioning the idea of mentalization here, I explore its relevance to emotions more fully in the second half of the book.

What follows are six vignettes that illustrate how identifying emotions manifests itself in psychotherapy. I am deliberately not dwelling on diagnosis as a way to affirm that the process of identifying emotions is relevant for many different kinds of patients. The first vignette involves a woman patient in her 40s, Amy, who reported being confused and uncertain about her reaction in hearing her boyfriend discuss the prospect of moving in together. Previously, they had talked about a plan to move in together, but on this occasion the boyfriend introduced the idea in terms of what he would do when his lease was up, emphasizing that he was definitely going to be moving. Amy had difficulty knowing what she felt in reaction. She knew it evoked something that had to do with trust and that she did not like it, but she had to search in order to further describe her reaction, which, it turned out, had to do with disappointment, tinged with anger. Both of Amy's parents had addiction problems, and she was sensitive about not being heard and being taken for granted. She experienced neglect, which would oscillate depending on her parents' demanding work schedules and large family gatherings. In addition to the impact of her family and personal history, there was a cultural aspect of Amy's experience: as an Asian woman, she felt an obligation to be discreet about her emotions if possible, not to make them explicitly known.

Amy's emotions would easily get lost and disappear even with her therapist, especially during the first 5 years of therapy. We had repeated interactions in which I would say, "I am not sure what's going on with you now," and she would respond with "I'm not sure either." A subsequent effort to figure it out was unlikely. However, with a bit of prompting from me—for example, "I wonder if you were more upset than you realized . . . ," she began to develop more of an interest in exploring her feelings.

Amy remained in therapy for a decade or so, and she grew much more comfortable acknowledging her feelings, apart from whether she wanted to express them. In the instance that I described with her boyfriend, our effort to identify her emotions helped her communicate with him. Interestingly, she did not disclose the intention to speak with her boyfriend in the session. She decided to do this on her own. The results were positive and mutually gratifying. Her boyfriend, who is also someone who often struggles to know what he feels, told her that he sees how his anxiety about the end of his lease led him to focus on his intentions in a way that left her out. He added that he could see why this would upset Amy, and he confirmed that what he really wanted was for them to move in together. Not all examples of identifying emotions bear such fruit, but in this case, Amy felt particularly proud of herself for overcoming the internalized expectation that she would endure but not express her feelings, and was delighted that her boyfriend acknowledged her feelings, as they were able to return to a path of moving ahead toward greater commitment. Amy used therapy well as a practice sphere to acknowledge her feelings in the world.

The second vignette involves a male patient in his late 20s, Bernardo, a tough guy you would not suspect was choosing to log time in therapy. Bernardo was not someone who had trouble knowing what he felt in the sense that he was often angry. He seemed to be angry about something in every session, and would readily report that others told him he was angry. Bernardo had been through anger management classes because of outbursts at work and had a history of physical altercations, including an awful knockdown battle with his father in the family kitchen when he was an adolescent. Bernardo was not motivated to talk much about his childhood, but from what I learned, he experienced opposing styles of parenting: aggressive discipline from his father and an absence of boundary setting (especially no disciplining) from his mother. Our work had three distinct elements: first, encouraging him to be aware of when he was becoming angry and to do some of the things he knew would help—like distracting himself and trying to calm down; second, encouraging him to tell me about what it meant for him to be angry; and third, wondering together about how his anger served as a kind of default emotion, which interfered with his comfortably being able to identify other emotions. It was interesting that until we worked on the second element, thinking about what anger meant, he had difficulty making progress with the first element, reducing the intensity of his anger.

I would like to be clear about what our work did and did not accomplish. Bernardo realized that he automatically felt that with anger, there was a kind of obligation to act. It never dawned on him that, given his family history, he could be angry and sit with that feeling, perhaps waiting until he was less angry and more ready to communicate his anger. He had some success with this, more in being able not to overreact to perceived slights (e.g., while driving, his "road rage" became something more like "road aggrieved") than in embodying wisdom and moderation. Bernardo was an intense person, and it is not likely that this personality trait would change. So, I cannot cite examples in which he would communicate his anger and have the kind of experience that Amy had in terms of receiving a response that made it easier to move beyond negative emotions. My efforts to encourage Bernardo to speculate about the mental states of others, which originally were met with a perplexed expression, started to bear fruit. Most significantly, our work helped Bernardo be aware of new emotions—his fear about whether his girl-friend would stick with the relationship, his joy to see that others seemed to be reacting differently to him at work and at play, and his sadness around his parents' aging and around his recognition that others had childhoods less filled with violent events and memories. The moments of sadness were brief, and fleeting, although meaningful.

The third vignette concerns a male patient in his 40s, Carlos, who came from a family in which emotions were expressed frequently and forcefully. Carlos understood his way of experiencing emotions as cul-turally normative for a Latino. Carlos was able to identify a wide range of emotions, but when agitated he was more imprecise, and therefore misleading in the way he described them. For example, when his wife became pregnant after a series of IVF (in vitro fertilization) failures, Carlos found himself easily upset, quickly perceiving the intentions of others as more deliberately negative than seemed warranted. So, he suspected that his doorman regarded him as having it easy because he worked from home, but he could cite no actual evidence that this was the case. Carlos was aware, too, that his reactivity was disturbing to his wife, and he was anxious about being hurtful to her and their baby. He was upset at making his wife upset, but he could not imagine what he might do to avoid doing this.

Our work centered on weighing what Carlos was feeling with more care and, with my encouragement, opting not to disclose what he was feeling to his wife. We actually rehearsed interactions in which he could practice responses that were not led by his emotions. This was extremely difficult for Carlos, and his first efforts were almost comical—he virtu-ally had to restrain himself from allowing his emotions to pour out. He improved over time, and in particular, it helped him to experience the emotion within himself, doing so fully, even if he was making the choice not to express it. It is interesting, furthermore, that Carlos felt positively about being able to stay with the emotion, rather than releas-ing it quickly.

The fourth vignette is about a woman in her late 30s, Deborah, with a vibrant career, a successful husband, and three children (a 16-year-old boy, a 12-year-old girl, and a 7-year-old boy). Deborah and her husband got along well for the most part: they shared similar values and enjoyed the company of many old, good friends. There was one area, however, in which they had repeated, frustrating conflict: over disciplining their children. Their older son, now 16, was not disciplined much, and Deb-orah's husband came to regret this and was determined to take more responsibility and action with the two younger children. Though Deborah was not fully on board with this, she seemed to go along with it but would interfere when she felt her husband was being too aggressive. For example, one day after school, their 12-year-old daughter said she was not feeling well and was too tired to clean up after dinner. Deborah's husband responded by ordering her to do it and, after some squabbling and crying, threatening not to allow her to have access to her cell phone. Deborah intervened and argued with her husband, starting a familiar, painful interaction between husband and wife, observed with distress by their daughter.

Deborah felt subtly intimidated by her husband and obliged to concur with his brand of discipline, and only half realized that, in fact, she disagreed with his ideas and had meaningful ideas of her own. This dynamic was fueled by the conversations that Deborah had with her husband in which he argued persuasively for his point of view and was dismissive of her attempts to articulate reasons that, as she saw it, disciplining rigidly was likely to be counterproductive. So, this was a situation in which Deborah knew and didn't know her own emotions: her frustration and anger came out in the heat of the moment, but there was an expectation that she ceded to, whereby these feelings would be displaced for the sake of marital harmony. Ironically, the effort to present a solid front with her husband backfired when their differences would explode in the presence of their daughter. Through therapy, Deborah began to appreciate that, for better or worse, she saw things differently from her husband, and that she had a right to these feelings. This was helpful to her, but her husband remained intransigent; so the conflict in the marriage remained unresolved. Our emotions are influenced by those around us, who can either be open and receptive, or not. Deborah's general inhibitory style was a factor in leading her to relinquish what she feels; over the course of therapy, she came to see how this pattern of behavior served her poorly. On her own, she realized that things were worse when she avoided her feelings.

The fifth vignette concerns a young man in his late teens, Ed, whose family was splitting apart just as he was embarking on leaving home. His family of origin was repressed, and information, especially emotionally laden information, like about the divorce, was not easy to come by. It was as if the family hired a therapist to be the repository of emotions from the patient in order for the parents to avoid dealing with the turmoil. Ed had been sent away to a boarding school but hated it, and his parents somewhat reluctantly allowed him to return home.

Ed and I would have the same interaction again and again, in which I would ask him to tell me how he felt, and he would proceed and tell me how he was supposed to feel. I would point this out to him, and he would seem mystified that I was asking for something that he simply felt aversive toward. For example, when he returned from the weekend when he visited his father in his new apartment in a far-flung suburb in New Jersey and I asked him, "So, how was it?" Ed responded by saying that "um . . . it all went as planned, the train was on time, the walk to the apartment complex was easy and quick, and it was really great to see the dog" (who, unlike Ed, was able to live in one place). I said something like "Great to see the dog, but what was it like to see Dad?" He replied, "Dad is Dad, he's always the same—we played tennis, went to his favorite new bar-restaurant, and then he asked me if I wanted to go to the movies, but I was tired and so we just went home." I said, "I feel like I am missing how you felt—was it weird? Was it fun? Was it sad?" Ed responded, "It was okay, it went okay, I know that Dad wanted me to come and I was glad I went . . . I mean the divorce was stressful for him, and he is just getting back on his feet in a new place, with a new life." This is an excellent example of how Ed was more comfortable focusing on his father's feelings than on his own. I surmised, from knowing him and the recent family history, that he must have some ambivalent feelings, and that he probably was sitting on some negative feelings about this visit. I was not sure, apart from what he had said, which obscured what he felt, if he was aware of other feelings. As best as I could tell, his feelings were aporetic, not formed clearly, with a hint of avoiding what he was uncomfortable facing. Ed was engaged in therapy and liked coming, but he was also happy to have the excuse to end it when his activities picked up at school. His capacity to identify emotions reminds us that this must exist on a continuum that is related to age. As a general rule, younger people are less adept at identifying emotions since they have had less practice doing so.

Our sixth vignette concerns about Franklin, a man in his mid-60s from a WASP background. This depiction is more complicated than the other five in this chapter, as I present something about his experience of emotions that has its source in my own emotional experience as a therapist. So, this is an instance of transaction in the emotional field and countertransference. My work with Franklin began with his realization that he was dangerously self-indulgent with various substances, and we had success in getting him to cease pot smoking and refrain from using sleeping pills every night. He had a number of concerns in coming to therapy, but addressing his concrete concerns first had the effect of making him feel better all around and supported a warm transference to me. His presentation was unruffled, but he was attentive and used language in a subtle, delightful way. Although we laughed and joked together easily, which usually would indicate a degree of comfort between us, I became aware that I felt anxious before our sessions and monitored the time throughout the session, which seemed to go slowly. I could identify my emotion as anxiety, but I could not make sense of why I would be feeling this emotion with this patient.

Was it possible that this was an example of projective identification? That I could use what I was feeling as a way to know what the patient was feeling but could not tolerate? Maybe; but maybe not. Franklin was a shrewd observer of himself and others. It was a pleasure to hear him elaborate on his feelings, and he even relished talking about the past, his family, and other formative relationships. He was in the process of rearranging his life: still occasionally working in his profession, but only selectively. He was motivated to talk about the present and the future as a way of figuring out how he wanted to spend his time. He was also motivated to engage in reflection about his life, which, he repeatedly emphasized, was, in fact, mostly lived. I know that I was struck by his frank acknowledgment about this notion of a "mostly lived" perspective on his life, as it challenged my naive expectation that he was coming to therapy because he wanted to change his life.

Perhaps one could speculate that my anxiety partly belonged to him but was partly my own. Our careers matched in terms of being in transition away from having greater formal responsibilities to fewer ones, with more freedom of choice but fewer day-to-day obligations. My experience was to be aware of feeling something, being confused about it, but able to imagine some of the forces that contributed to it. It helped the treatment in the sense that beyond his smooth self-presentation, he was worried about the next phase of life.

These six vignettes show various aspects of identifying emotions. They are not offered as constituting a comprehensive account. Indeed, they are arbitrary in the sense that there are many others that I might have presented. With Amy, we encounter someone who is confused and unsure of what she feels, but therapy helps her beyond this. With Bernardo, we meet someone who seems like he knows what he feels—namely, anger—and readily acts on it, but who comes to appreciate how he uses anger to obscure other emotions. With Carlos, we also have someone who assumes that if one feels something, action is the immediate result, but who learns that it can be desirable to sit longer with an emotion. With Deborah, we hear about a person who is conflicted, who knows and does not know what she feels, and who moves from being absorbed with the emotion of the other to owning her own feelings. With Ed, we are introduced to an adolescent who adopts a strategy of feeling what he should feel and thereby loses touch with what he actually feels. With Franklin, we consider how a therapist's emotion leads to understanding the patient's emotion, which was on the fringe of the patient's awareness.

These vignettes concern a range of patients. One feature of all of them is the patient's aporetic emotions. This is demonstrated in how Amy was confused, Bernardo obscured other emotions besides anger, Carlos became vague when aroused, Deborah experienced conflict, Ed dismissed his own emotions, and Franklin kept his anxiety distant from his awareness. It is apparent that while aporetic emotions can define one's initial experience, they can occur later in the process of identifying emotions as well. Not all emotions follow a trajectory from being unknown to becoming known. Emotions can come in and out of focus, and that is why the task of identifying emotions is more complex and daunting than it might seem.

In this chapter, I have been concerned with the challenge of identifying emotions. Difficulty in identifying emotions is something we all experience, although it can be an indication of more pervasive psychopathology. Failure to be able to identify emotions is one of three factors in determining alexithymia, and alexithymia has been correlated with several different kinds of psychopathology. Whether a patient can or cannot identify emotions is crucial, telling information, and besides an evaluation of risk factors, it is the first thing that I try to assess with new patients. However, identifying emotions is not just relevant to psychotherapeutic process; it is a phenomenon of everyday life, and part of how we communicate with others.

The example from Sarah Silverman enables us to glimpse a subtle aspect of identifying emotions. As an adolescent she is immersed in fear, in the context of being depressed and traumatized, but as an adult, she manages to use her suffering to tame the influence of her emotions—not to give them up, but to acquire enough distance so that they can be incorporated into humor, connecting her to others, and more lovingly to herself. Here we are on the edges of identifying emotions, where we need to begin to think about modulating emotions.

Our clinical examples demonstrate that therapy might involve coming to name emotions as well as to make sense of what they mean. Aporetic emotions are common, and even where it seems that one knows what one feels, there can be self-deception. To some extent, identifying emotions requires that one can sustain the experience of emotions; however, it might also support the relinquishing of an emotion, depending on the context. Linehan (Linehan & Wilks, 2015) offers the helpful notion that identifying emotions can include describing them. Yet, as I have observed, identifying emotions has become more challenging in a postmodern society in which we cannot assume that a consensus exists about their meaning. Identifying emotions will be affected by one's personal history (development), one's family life, and one's culture or ethnicity. A culture in which one is obliged to grab a sword if insulted is very different from a culture in which to be civilized is to not reveal one's true feelings.

Ultimately, identifying emotions is a first step in the process of experiencing emotions. It is a necessary but insufficient condition for using emotions well. I do not think it is impossible to act on an emotion without identifying it. However, it is most often the case that either one does know what one feels or at least that one has some idea. In the face of having aporetic emotions, it is natural to imagine that one would seek to identify them. This can be fairly easy or it can be painful and elusive, requiring lots of effort. As psychodynamic therapists know, reducing the mystery of aporetic emotions can take multiple explorations over a long period of time.

Identifying emotions only takes us so far in our journey. As we move in the direction of fathoming emotional experience, we are entering the terrain of modulating emotions. Indeed, we ought to keep in mind that the distinction between identifying and modulating emotions is designed to help mental health professionals work effectively with emotion. With that in mind, let us take the next step and take account of the modulation of emotions.

 CHAPTER 2

Modulating Emotions

We can educate our emotions but not suppress them
entirely, and the feelings we have inside are a testimony to
our lack of success.
—ANTONIO R. DAMASIO, *The Feeling
of What Happens* (1999)

With modulation, we are moving into the realm of how we value emotions. Valuing depends on a sense of agency, although this does not have to mean conscious agency. Modulating emotions is a step beyond identifying emotions, away from aporetic emotions, and toward greater specificity. Modulating emotions overlaps with one of the most important recent constructs in the study of emotion, namely emotion regulation. My reasons for preferring the term "modulating" over "regulating" will be established later in the chapter, but briefly let me say that they are based on the etymology and connotations of the respective words as well as on substance. Regulation is related to control and fits models where cognition subdues emotion, whereas modulation is related to music (like varying tone, pitch, or strength of voice or note; like changing key) and also science (like varying amplitude, frequency, or other characteristic of a wave or signal). Modulation connotes being responsive, making adjustments, and making efforts to blend and join together important aspects of how emotions can be valued and revalued.

Identifying emotions typically is the prelude to modulating emotions. As we have observed, though, identifying emotions can extend to trying to make sense of their meaning, not just naming them, which makes the distinction between identifying and modulating emotions murky. Modulating emotions means processing them, rather than just experiencing them. There is not much research on the distinction between identifying and modulating emotions, but one interesting study concluded that cognitive reappraisal, the basic mechanism of emotion regulation (modulation), is a more effective strategy than labeling emotions; intriguingly, however, the subjects imagined that labeling would not decrease distress, although, in fact, it did so (Lieberman, Inagaki, Tabibnia, & Crockett, 2011). This finding supports the notion that identifying emotions can be underestimated in importance and that modulating emotions is a potentially even more valuable strategy.

Before discussing emotion regulation, I would like to begin by describing a fundamental contrast in theorizing about emotions, which bears on our potential for regulation of emotions. This contrast is between the Aristotelian and the Stoic approach, which I have elaborated on previously in Chapter 2 of *Affect Regulation, Mentalization, and the Development of the Self* (Fonagy et al., 2002). Aristotelians are committed to the potential of educating our emotions through practice so that they occur in the right way, at the right time, to the right people. Stoics, on the contrary, believe our emotions, by definition, are overpowering, and that the best we can do is to distance ourselves from acting under their influence. Hybrid perspectives have been articulated: for example, Spinoza largely follows the Stoics but emphasizes the importance of understanding emotions, even if they are dangerous to act upon.

The literature on emotion regulation clearly comes down on the Aristotelian side. Our potential to modulate and refine our emotional responses affirms the idea that emotions are not by definition overwhelming and unruly. However, questions about limits to regulating emotions are not often acknowledged in the literature on emotion regulation, and I return to this issue again in the chapter. With this brief historical sketch in mind, let us introduce an autobiographical example before turning to examine contemporary theories and research about emotion regulation.

LOSS AND LOVE: TRACY K. SMITH

Tracy K. Smith's (2015) memoir, *Ordinary Light*, portrays a young, African American woman coming to terms with her mother's death. Her emotions are portrayed subtly and wisely—she refers to a youthful experience of fear by speculating, "In fear, isn't there often an undetected tinge of fantasy" (p. 178). The story begins with her mother's death scene and then moves back in time, narrating her own development and ending with a return to coping with her grief. Smith seems to be suggesting that we could not understand what her mother's death means to her without delving into how her own history and personality were formed by this relationship.

Smith's autobiographical tale traces her evolution from co-regulation with her mother to self-regulation, which we witness by appreciating the extent to which her mourning is guided by the power of her mother's love. Self-regulation is an achievement, and accompanied inevitably with some pain. Yet, self-regulation can exist and be sustained only by means of co-regulation, which recedes but never simply disappears. Smith's mother is consistently portrayed as a loving, admirable, and pious woman who holds the family together through her devout faith, but who always manages to be "mirthsome" (p. 58). As the youngest of seven children, Smith grows up in a loving family, which she affectionately characterizes as "an invincible unit" (p. 28).

Smith recounts the pleasure of togetherness that she experienced with her mother in luxurious detail—for example, listening to her mother read a religious book for children: "As my mother read, I'd sometimes let my eyes drift across her face, taking her in out of habit, memorizing her, breathing in her smell, the way she held herself, the lilting cadence of her voice" (p. 17). Another example occurs after a disappointing experience bobbing for apples at a Halloween party, which Smith's mother helped to organize, even though her mother was ambivalent for religious reasons about celebrating such a pagan holiday. A wonderful moment of modulating emotions in an upward direction occurs on their drive home:

> . . . watching her hands calm yet firm upon the wheel and the way she looked down at me from time to time, letting me smile up into her face and returning the smile with real warmth, with love I could see and feel—I could tell that no matter what she believed in, right at the very moment she and I were alone together, Kathy and Tracy, just our two souls in the car moving surely toward home, full and intact with something bigger and more real than any of the questions or beliefs we might struggle to fit into words. I knew, just at that very moment, that she was glad in the way every mother who makes her child happy is glad. (p. 32)

Although this example of togetherness is from Smith's point of view, it is striking how she recognizes her mother here as well as feels recognized by her. The experience, it seems, is mutual.

During adolescence, Smith begins to retreat within, and grows apart from her mother. This happens as Smith questions the kind of religion practiced by her mother and is spurred by an unconsummated "affair" with a teacher at school. Smith tells us about awakening from a dream around this time: "In the dark center of night, hours from dawn, I'd lie still in bed, stranded, caught between competing currents of feeling: disbelief that salvation could really be as literal as all that and a strange, powerful nostalgia for the very years I was in the process of living, when the world of my family was the only heaven I needed to believe in" (p. 125). Smith distances herself further from her family when she moves from Northern California, where she had grown up, to attend Harvard. As she avers: "I let my own wishes and desires replace the values that she sought to instill in me. But if I really felt that way, why didn't I ever tell her so?" (p. 241).

Smith makes the choice not to confront her mother with their differences, but this does not mean they are not apparent between them. A current of their old relationship coexists with a new degree of estrangement. Indeed, Smith acknowledges with painful candor, in the context of angrily arguing with her father after her mother's death, "I'd never spoken so freely or so honestly with my mother. I'd never had the occasion, having hidden from her everything that would have brought our most starkly differing viewpoints into contact" (p. 331).

Yet, this is not the whole story. However much Smith documents her skepticism of her mother's religiosity, and how they grew apart, she also discloses how her mother lives within her as a benevolent presence. In a moving, sweet, and sad moment before her mother dies, angels come to her mother and forecast that Smith will become a writer (p. 318). Moreover, after her mother's death, Smith comes to the realization that there might be something about her love of poetry that was similar to what her mother experienced through prayer (p. 311).

Smith's memoir is the story of her love for her mother and her mourning for her premature death (at 58 years old, when Smith was 22 years old), intertwined with a coming-of-age tale. We come to know Smith through the lens of her mother's death. The memoir ends with a vivid memory/fantasy of being 3 years old: Smith is snuggling with her mother and conveys an exquisite sense of comfort. She says, "Mommy?" Her mother replies, "Yes, Tracy." And Tracy utters," "Oh, nothing . . . nothing" (p. 349). Co-regulation, deeply connected, Smith unabashedly feels herself as her mother's daughter. This saga is relevant to the subject of modulating emotions because it shows us someone who endures the emotional pain of losing a loved one, but who can handle it precisely because of her mother's love. Smith admires her mother, without idealizing her, which is particularly apparent in reflecting on her mother's history as an African-American woman born in Alabama (who participated in the civil rights movement). Smith offers us an intimate sense of what it feels like to grieve: a process, a convoluted one, and one that is powerfully influenced by early life development. This journey of modulating emotions is long and slow; it changes, but it does not come to an end.

MODELS OF EMOTION REGULATION: COGNITIVE PROCESSING

No topic in psychology has generated more widespread and growing interest than emotion regulation, and no topic has greater potential to be a unifying force across so many domains of knowledge within psychology—clinical, developmental, cognitive, neuropsychology, social and personality, diversity, physiological, addiction, and experimental—and among related fields like the neurosciences, the social sciences, and philosophy. The proliferating interest in emotion regulation is documented in Figure 2.1.

Yet, writing about emotion regulation is an elusive and complicated business. No consensus exists about the range of phenomena that it entails, despite the emergence of more complex models (Aldao, 2012; Gross, 2008, Cole, Martin, & Dennis, 2004; Gratz & Roemer, 2004; Gross & Thompson, 2007; Koole, 2009; Mennin & Fresco, 2009; Waters et al., 2010). I begin by describing the process model of emotion regulation, a promising model that relies on the notion of cognitive

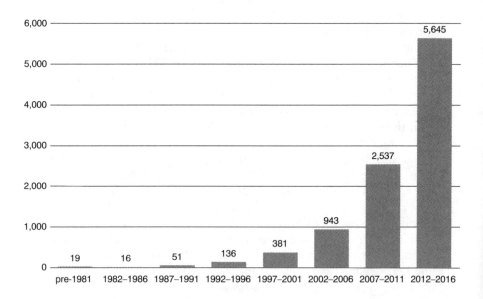

FIGURE 2.1. Proliferating references to "emotion regulation." References in PsycINFO, pre-1981 to 2016.

reappraisal, and then move on in the next section to the mindfulness model, which represents a critique of the process model, emphasizing acceptance over the transformation of emotions. I provide some reasons to defend a different model that is based on development and, in Part II, I sketch out my alternative, which emphasizes the relation between mentalizing emotion and the self. I affirm that the self can be used as the means through which emotions are regulated, but concur with those who see emotion regulation as part of self-regulation (Baumeister, Zell, & Tice, 2007; Koole, 2009). As we have seen in the example from Smith, not only is early development crucial as an influence on self-regulation, but co-regulation does not disappear and coexists with self-regulation. Later in this book, I shall defend a model that is based on "mentalized affectivity," an aspect of emotion regulation that it is not merely an online event, but is influenced by autobiographical memory (AM), which is a fundamental part of being, having, and cultivating a sense of self.

Gross and Thompson's (2007) process model of emotion regulation is impressive in its scope, delineating several parts of an online process, anchored by cognitive reappraisal. As this model depicts it, emotion regulation involves various strategies, whereby various temporal possibilities are carefully articulated. Five distinct processes are described and elaborated upon: situation selection, situation modification, attentional deployment, cognitive change, and response modulation. These five processes are understood as "families" in that they are related but distinct. A key distinction is made between processes that are antecedent focused—that is, the first four above—and response modulation, the last one, which is response focused. Recursion in emotion is shown using a feedback loop in the model in Figure 2.2.

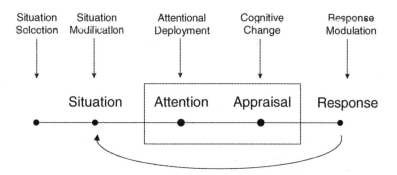

FIGURE 2.2. Recursion in emotion shown using a feedback loop in the process model. From Gross and Thompson (2007, p. 10). Copyright © 2007 The Guilford Press. Reprinted by permission.

Situation selection involves taking actions that make it more (or less) likely that we will end up in a situation we expect will give rise to desirable (or undesirable) emotions. It is forward looking, leading us to weigh short-term versus longer-term benefits. Examples of situation selection include avoiding an offensive coworker, watching a funny movie after a bad day, seeking out a friend with whom we can have a good cry. These examples converge around the attempt to minimize the expected experience of negative emotions, but there is no reason not to imagine how this might work with positive emotions such as canceling a meeting in order to spend more time with your grandchild.

Situation modification means making direct efforts to change situations. Gross and Thompson (2007) point out that this is a mainstay of parenting, and their examples underscore this: helping your child with a frustrating puzzle or setting up an elaborate doll tea party. Situation modification, as they describe it, bears a close connection to socialization. Gross and Thompson observe that it is hard to draw a clear line between situation selection and modification, as the latter itself can call a new situation into being. They also acknowledge that what they are describing is extrinsic: "Also, although we have previously emphasized that situations can be external or internal, situation modification—as we mean it here—has to do with modifying external, physical environments" (p. 12).

The next process in the unfolding of emotion regulation is attentional deployment, wherein an emotion is regulated through a shift in attention, without changing the environment. Gross and Thompson understand attention deployment as an inward version of situation selection. Attention deployment relies on two specific strategies: distraction and concentration. With distraction, our attention shifts from one thing to another; with concentration, our attention zeroes in on something for a closer examination. An example of the former occurs when one invokes thoughts or memories that are inconsistent with an undesirable emotional state; an example of the latter is rumination. Rumination is a tricky example of concentration, as it is typically used to convey a kind of attention that is stuck, and thus inadvertently raises the question of being a strategy that is not optimal and may even be pathological.

The fourth process is cognitive change, which arguably is the most important part of the model, as it reveals the extent to which regulation depends on an integration of emotion and cognition. Cognitive change refers to altering the appraisal of the situation we are in to amend its emotional significance, either by changing how we think about the situation or about our capacity to manage the demands it poses. Gross and Thompson introduce the phenomenon of "downward social comparison" as an example, whereby we help ourselves to feel better by comparing our situation to those of others who are even more unfortunate. Cognitive change entails a reappraisal in the sense that we revise the original appraisal that forms the occurrence of the emotion itself.

The fifth and final process is response modulation, which sequentially occurs late in process. Response modulation can influence many different aspects of response: physiological, experiential, or behavioral. Commonly, response modulation is manifest in the expression, or suppression, of emotion. However, response modulation might include using drugs, eating, or exercising. Its proper aim, according to Gross and Thompson, is adaptation, like problem solving or interpersonal understanding, as opposed to mere venting. Context, therefore, is important: a toddler's crying can be adaptive in some circumstances, less so in others.

Gross and Thompson's process model of emotion regulation covers a lot of ground, and their distinction between antecedent-focused and response-focused regulation is illuminating in clarifying how emotions prompt us to initiate various actions. Yet, as Loewenstein (2007) points out, it is open to question whether situation selection or response modulation genuinely belong to regulation, as they appear to produce alternative directions that serve to preclude the effort to mediate emotions. Gross and Thompson seem to demonstrate the point that not all emotions are or need to be regulated. However, they mainly follow the arc of possible scenarios once an emotion occurs, emphasizing how it is altered

Let us reflect on some of the assumptions and implications of Gross and Thompson's perspective. First, the process model of emotion regulation, like stress models, which predate it, bears the mark of its origins in engineering. The human organism strives to return to a state of equilibrium, or homeostasis, and deviations from homeostasis, especially long-lasting ones, wreak havoc on the system. The process model relies on stimulus–response, where an organism makes adjustments in reaction to (or in anticipation of) events in the external environment. Though they acknowledge the possibility of internal stimulus, they do not grant it much attention.

The focus of the process model is weighted to individual experience. Yet, most of Gross and Thompson's examples actually involve others, which raises important questions about shared or intersubjective aspects of emotion regulation, which we have observed so poignantly in Smith's memoir. Campos and colleagues (2011, 2003) have voiced concern that most research on emotion regulation uses the paradigm of a single individual, whereas in real life, it is more likely that emotions are regulated in relation to others. There are, I believe, two reasons for this bias: first, the valorization of individualism and the desirability of dealing with things on one's own in Western culture; and second, the model's mechanistic origin, which, on the one hand, makes it parsimonious, but, on the other hand, means that valuable intrapersonal and interpersonal subtleties are obscured.

Subsequent research that focuses on cognitive reappraisal has raised questions about its effectiveness. For example, Webb, Miles, and Sheeran's (2012) meta-analysis of emotion regulation strategies suggested that "cognitive change" had only a small-to-medium effect, whereas, surprisingly, distraction was effective. Webb and colleagues also show that reappraising the emotional response proved less effective than reappraising the emotional stimulus. Another recent study suggests that cognitive reappraisal is often overlooked as an emotion regulation strategy: only 16% of subjects used cognitive reappraisal as a response to a negatively valenced image, even where a follow-up option was possible (Suri, Whittaker, & Gross, 2015). The authors conclude that context must play an important role, as even in a follow up study, they were able to increase reappraisal when the default options were removed.

Finally, the process model leaves much for us to wonder about concerning human agency: Who and what is at the source of cognitive appraisals? Where would we locate the sense of self? To what extent and how do personality style/traits as well as personal histories have an impact on emotion regulation? If emotions are mostly seen as indicators of a system that needs rebalancing, the sense of self becomes a remote consideration.

MODELS OF EMOTION REGULATION: MINDFULNESS

An alternative perspective on emotion regulation has been put forth in the expanding literature of mindfulness. In this section, I shall examine some recent work that applies the theory of mindfulness to emotion regulation, especially where it has begun to be studied empirically. The mindfulness model is mainly theoretical, though, and it has a clinical and health psychology bent.

In attempting to delineate the mechanisms of mindfulness, Shapiro and her colleagues (Shapiro, Carlson, Astin, & Freedman, 2006) have reformulated mindfulness in terms of the notion of "reperceiving." As they understand it, reperceiving is a meta-mechanism that grants perspective: "Rather than being immersed in the drama of our personal narrative or life story, we are able to stand back and simply witness it" (p. 377). Reperceiving has three intersecting components: intention, attention, and attitude.

Shapiro's understanding of "intention" links it to the Buddhist focus on enlightenment and compassion for all things. Its goal is not just self-regulation, but self-exploration and self-liberation. "Attention" is defined in terms of the capacity to observe the operations of one's moment-to-moment internal and external experience, and, more specifically, the ability to attend for long periods of time to one object (vigilance or sustained attention); the ability to shift the focus of attention between objects at will (switching); and the ability to inhibit secondary elaborative processing of thoughts, feelings, and sensations (cognitive inhibition). In describing "attitude," Shapiro notes that the literal translation of mindfulness in Japanese is "heartmindfulness." She elaborates attitude to mean attending to one's own experience "without evaluating or interpretation;" and, more specifically, to mean curiosity and taking interest in things, but also allowing them to pass away—"the capacity not to continually strive for pleasant experiences, or to push aversive experiences away" (p. 377).

Shapiro and colleagues make a number of strong claims about reperceiving as a process: that it allows the subject to see him or herself as an object; that it increases the capacity for objectivity about one's own internal experience; that it expands the capacity to take the perspective of another; and that it fosters empathy, not detachment, apathy, or numbness. Reperceiving is a way to choose what has previously been reflexively adopted or conditioned. The authors also suggest a link between reperceiving and the idea of "decentering" used in mindfulness-based cognitive therapy.

The mindfulness model represents a contrast, and to some extent, a challenge to the process model. Where the process model presumes that emotion regulation is situational, the mindfulness model highlights that it can be reflective. The former is based on stimulus-response but does not exclude internal experience; while the latter tunes in to internal experience but does not exclude external experience. So, emotion regulation ought not be conceived exclusively as an online phenomenon because it involves the reprocessing of experience as well. Nevertheless, some views of mindfulness, which are conceived in terms of meditational practices, affirm the idea of mindfulness as dwelling in the present, that is, avoiding preoccupation with the past or the future, and redirecting attention back to the present moment (Feldman, Hayes, Kumar, Greeson, & Laurenceau, 2007).

Moreover, there is a significant difference in emphasis between the process model, which features the transformation of emotion through regulation, and the mindfulness model, which features the idea of accepting emotions. As Erisman and Roemer (2010) maintain, "Instead of attempting to change or alter emotional experiences, a mindful stance toward emotional experiences would involve noticing and observing emotions simply as they are and bringing compassion and acceptance to emotional reactions as they arise" (p. 72). Farb and colleagues (2010) are explicit in questioning the centrality of cognitive appraisal: "A plausible mechanism of action for mindfulness effects may include the development of metacognitive skills for detached viewing of emotions, rather than the elaboration of emotional content through cognitive reappraisal" (p. 31).

Shapiro's notion of reperceiving has the connotation of preserving the experience of emotions, not exercising control over the emotion. Some views of mindfulness countenance more of an active stance than others, while others emphasize that the meaning of acceptance must be restricted to the absence of evaluation. Hayes and Plumb (2007) propose, for example, that acceptance is not an end in itself, suggesting that it is a way to generate values-based action. However, it remains to be clarified, even if we consider acceptance as a means, how it translates into well-being.

Chambers, Gullone, and Allen (2009) have argued that it is important to distinguish mindfulness as a construct, practice, or process in the context of postulating that mindfulness and emotion regulation might be integrated as "mindful emotion regulation." They distinguish between more cognitive approaches to mindfulness, where the emphasis is on a nonelaborative awareness of the present moment (and avoiding secondary processes), and practices such meditation that aim for personal and spiritual progress. Citing Siegel (2007), they describe how mindfulness can be understood as altering "the relationship individuals have toward their mental processes" (p. 562). From this perspective, "mindfulness can be understood to promote personal autonomy—that is, to enhance the individual's capacity to act in accord with their personal interests . . . rather than being driven by self-relevant cognition" (Brown, Ryan, & Creswell, 2007, p. 563). Ultimately, Chambers, Gullone, and Allen observe that mindfulness is an antithetical strategy to emotion suppression, the latter of which is less adaptive than cognitive reappraisal, as Gross (2006) has argued, and they propose that while cognitive reappraisal is antecedently focused on content, mindfulness should be valued as a process that encourages us to accept, and not necessarily to act on, emotions and thoughts (p. 566, 569).

It is worth pondering the ambiguity concerning mindfulness and the role of the self. On the one hand, mindfulness is regarded as preventing us from being self-immersed, expressly aiding us in overcoming the danger of self-involvement; on the other hand, Shapiro and colleagues (2006) and Chambers and colleagues (2009) urge us to appreciate that mindfulness contributes to the enhancement of the capacity to observe the self. Clearly, mindfulness advocates value self-control, but they also value being able to leave the self behind. Brown and colleagues (2007) see mindfulness as challenging the "primacy of the ego" and as requiring a "disengagement from self-concern," but they end up averring—without explanation—that it fosters a "more fundamental 'I'." Davidson (2010) provides a revealing gloss on this point: "Mindfulness training can be hypothesized to change an individual's relationship to his or her emotions so that they are not viewed as fundamental constituents of self, but rather as more fleeting phenomena that appear to the self" (p. 10).

Ambiguity about the self, however, is not something that pertains just to mindfulness—all therapies have to grapple with whether they help us realize or transcend the self. Indeed, ambiguity about the self is deeply ingrained in our culture, however much Western culture is typically seen as affirming the value of autonomous selfhood. What does it mean that we have the words "selfish" and "selfless," but not a word for the right amount of being concerned with oneself—what psychoanalysts refer to as "healthy narcissism"?

EMOTION REGULATION IN DEVELOPMENT: ATTACHMENT, MENTALIZATION, AND THE SELF

Human beings are not born with the capacity to regulate their emotions. Infants learn to regulate their emotions through a natural process of maturation of the brain and with considerable help from primary caregivers. Indeed, the function of the attachment system is to promote the reliance of infants on their caregivers, so that co-regulation can facilitate the emergence of self-regulation. The capacity for emotion regulation unfolds as a biological function, incorporating temperament as well as the input from the attachment relationship between caregivers and infant. Secure attachment produces a healthy and flexible form of emotion regulation, while insecure attachment produces less than optimal styles (avoidant insecure producing an overregulation of emotion; preoccupied insecure producing an underregulation of emotions), and disorganized attachment produces an unpredictable and least effective form. Consequently, the ability/inability to regulate emotions determines one's sense of efficacy and agency, which parenthetically has implications for psychopathology, especially for the emergence of depression (MacLeod & Bucks, 2011; Williams et al., 2007).

Calkins and Hill (2007) venture the powerful claim that emotion regulation is the "critical achievement of early childhood" (p. 231). They emphasize the evolution from passive to active during the second year of life, where infants gain better control of their levels of arousal. Calkins and Hill demonstrate that secure infants who are able to make use of social referencing and express a need for social intervention are on the path to regulating their emotions effectively, whereas insecure avoidant infants rely on self-soothing and solitary exploration, which, in the long run, prove to be ineffective strategies. They also note that attachment style predicts how infants regulate negative affect in contexts beyond the specific activation of attachment. So, there are more general implications concerning emotion regulation from attachment that are not restricted to the attachment relationships per se.

According to Calkins and Hill (2007), attachment processes can impact emotion regulation in several ways: (1) affecting the development and functioning of physiological processes; (2) predicting specific emotional responses in the context of the relationship dyad itself, observable in the interactions between caregiver and infant; and (3) fostering the development and use of specific strategies outside the context of the attachment relationship that call for a more independent regulation of emotion (p. 243). Calkins and Hill stress that emotion regulation is best accounted for in terms of the larger construct of self-regulation, but they do not focus on the convoluted relation among attachment, emotion regulation, and the self.

To better understand how emotion regulation fosters the sense of self, we turn to Gergely's biosocial feedback theory (Fonagy et al., 2002; Gergely, 2007; Gergely & Unoka, 2008; Gergely & Watson, 1996). Gergely offers a complex portrait of the emergence of the self that is related to emotion regulation. The infant's sense of self, he asserts, is transformed from being "invisible" to "visible" through "affective mirroring." In this account, affect mirroring derives from contingency in infant learning and the acquisition of the "intentional stance," wherein infants 9–12 months old, but not 6-month-old infants, can interpret another as goal oriented and, in fact, can predict his or her future action toward goals in a new situation.

According to Gergely (2007), emotions are our earliest mental states, consisting of prewired bidirectional connections between facial expression and corresponding physiological states that are active from birth. Infants are not yet sensitive to the internal state cues that indicate basic emotions at birth, although a strong biosocial preparedness soon begins to emerge. Toward the end of the first year of life, Gergely claims, infants achieve a new level of emotional awareness and control that goes along with a better understanding of and reasoning about the feeling states of others. Regulation occurs only when secondary control structures have been created, encoding the meaning of infants' basic emotions. Mirroring produces these secondary representations in a causal sense—by means of a feedback process that sensitizes and increases internal control. Through the mechanisms of contingency detection and maximizing, the infant experiences causal efficacy as well as positive affect.

A sense of the self as agent unfolds through this process. Mirroring is distinct from an activity like soothing, wherein an infant's state is changed without necessarily contributing to his or her sense of agency. In affective mirroring, the caregiver reflects the infant's state back to the infant in a "marked" way. The marked quality differentiates the affect as belonging to the infant, rather than to the caregiver. The caregiver's expression of affect here is an imperfect exaggeration of the infant's state. As Gergely (2007) proposes, the infant "decouples" the affect from belonging to the caretaker and then "anchors" it to him- or herself. In more recent work, Gergely (Gergely & Unoka, 2008) adds that the infant acquires the "pedagogical stance," which renders him or her to be receptive to parental input. The pedagogical stance means that the infant develops an interrogatory mode that transcends the motivation of safety that defines the attachment relationship; parental input serves to provide the groundwork for the infant to develop a sense of self, but also to be able to trust in order to keep learning and be able to modulate emotions in a culturally appropriate way.

Affect mirroring helps the infant gain crucial developmental functions, having to do with state regulation, the establishment of secondary representations that become associated with primary affect states (enhancing the cognitive capacity to access and attribute affects to the self), and the development of a generalized communicative code characterized by decoupling, anchoring, and the suspension of realistic consequences. The last function relates to the unfolding of the pedagogical stance and is also the basis for the emergent capacity to engage in imaginary play. Through affect mirroring, the sense of self evolves, so the infant becomes invested in heeding and utilizing subjective experience.

Related to the pedagogical stance, Gergely and colleagues have proposed the notion that it is valuable for infants to develop "epistemic trust" (Gergely, 2013; Gergely, Egyed, & Király, 2007; see also Koenig & Harris, 2005). Epistemic trust denotes that infants rely on caregivers to learn and become acculturated beings. It comes into being through ostensive cues such as eye contact, turn taking, and a special tone of voice. Without epistemic trust, infants are forced prematurely to rely on themselves and, as I discuss later in the book, a lack of epistemic trust can lead to psychopathology and poor responsiveness in psychotherapy. Epistemic vigilance, which emerges at 3–5 years old, is important as young children discern that not everyone is trustworthy, and so they need to be able to assess the reliability of the information they receive. Both epistemic trust and epistemic vigilance contribute to the capacity to modulate emotions: the former assuring co-regulation, the latter fostering self-regulation.

Neurobiological accounts dovetail with Gergely's account, especially concerning specifics about the emergence of the sense of self. Following the work of Hofer (1990), Schore (1994, 2003) supports the notion of a biology of attachment, such that the external regulation of the caregiver determines the neurochemistry of the infant's brain and hence his or her own regulation. Schore (1994) asserts that the infant's interactions with the caregiver "directly elicit psychoendocrinological changes that influence the biochemical activation of gene-action systems which program the critical period growth and differentiation of a corticolimbic structure responsible for self-regulation" (p. 18). At the beginning of life, the infants are immersed in achieving biological regulation, in particular, regulating levels of arousal with a stress on limiting the force of negative affect. Toward the end of the first year, according to Schore, the prefrontal cortex matures, which causes the mother's role to shift from being an "auxiliary cortex" to becoming a socializing agent as the infant provides regulation for him- or herself.

By the end of the first year of life, the prefrontal cortex begins to play a more active role in the modulation of affects. Activation of the prefrontal cortex coincides with an enhanced capacity for positive affect; thus, regulation modulates both negative and positive affect. Also around the end of the first year of life, the infant develops a greater ability to have delayed responses, which augments the range of possible reactions. In the second year of life, infants become more social, and new affects emerge. A particular focus for Schore is the appearance of the affect of shame, which develops between 14 and 16 months; shame exemplifies the dawning of self-consciousness—that one grasps oneself as an agent from an objective, not merely subjective stance (see Leary, 2007, too, on this point). At 18 months, a number of other dramatic events occur: as the infant is introduced to new forms of socialization, the caregiver is no longer merely a voice of positive affect, but also a voice of instruction and direction. The infant is now encouraged to be able to tolerate frustration and to opt for delayed gratification, as he or she learns that "good things come to those who wait." During this period, the caregiver's reaction to the infant's frustration is instrumental in determining whether it becomes an acceptable emotion or a "not-me" experience that needs to be thwarted or eliminated. If the latter is the case, shame comes to accompany later experiences of frustration.

What it means to be a self, therefore, significantly shifts at 18 months. Schore maintains that one's representational world undergoes a change at this time: from presymbolic representations, which encode the physiological–affective responses to the expressive face of the attachment figure, to symbolic representations, which are internalizations of the child's affect and the caregiver's response and are accessible to modulate distress-related affects. He argues that the core of the self lies in patterns of affect regulation that integrate the sense of self across state transitions, creating a continuity of inner experience. Emotion regulation lies at the basis of the self, but the development of the self has an influence on what it means to regulate emotions, rendering us capable of more subtle and precise responses. Schore's work is consistent with Lewis (2011) in showing that self-awareness can be discerned through visual self-recognition, the use of personal pronouns (like "me" and "mine"), and pretend play, and that it is necessary in order for self-conscious emotions—as opposed to basic emotions—to emerge.

Howe and Courage (1997) also describe the emergence of a new sense of self—which they term the "cognitive self" at 18–24 months, arguing that it coincides with the capacity for AM. Others, like Nelson and Fivush (2004), do not accept Howe and Courage's argument about children's use of AM, maintaining that it occurs much later. There is a consensus, though, that children only gradually become able to apprehend their emotional responses in light of their knowledge of themselves and their history.

The ability for children to see their emotions as part of their psychological makeup is developed through multiple interactions in which others interpret their internal states, and they attempt to interpret the others' states as well. Fonagy and colleagues (2002) describe this process as "mentalization." The concept has diverse origins, which is described in some detail in Chapter 4, and can be defined as the capacity to read and interpret mental states. Fonagy and colleagues added a focus on emotions, using ideas from attachment theory and psychoanalysis, to the mainly cognitive focus in the cognitive sciences. Mentalization unfolds from development, where being mentalized about (by others) spurs the evolution of mentalizing (by the self). It has an inherent basis in emotional experience as it occurs within the context of the attachment relationship, and it pertains to one's relationship to oneself, not just to others.

There is disagreement about when mentalization emerges developmentally, and whether its trajectory is separate from attachment and emotion regulation. No one would dispute that there is a progressive capacity to understand the mental states of others as mental states, and that the skill that evolves at 3–4 years old is necessary for more complex forms of emotion regulation. Gergely and Jacob (2012) note that by 3–4 years old, children have a greater capacity to use and comprehend language and to inhibit their impulses. Sperber and colleagues (2010) propose that epistemic trust is supplemented by epistemic vigilance around this same time. Indeed, as Heyes and Frith (2014) argue, the neural systems implicated in mind reading are the last to reach maturity and continue to develop from adolescence to adulthood. So, there is a long developmental story concerning mentalization, and the relationship between mentalization and emotion regulation, that we are just beginning to understand.

MEASURES OF EMOTION REGULATION

Various measures of emotion regulation have been introduced that focus on the construct in general, but also on how it can be utilized as a tool in diagnosing and assessing psychopathology. In this section, I select three measures for discussion (and do not make an effort to provide a comprehensive account): (1) the Difficulties in Emotion Regulation Scale (DERS), (2) the Emotion Regulation Questionnaire (ERQ), and (3) the Affective Style Questionnaire (ASQ). There are many other emotion regulation scales, but these three have contributed to our understanding of the concept and are relevant to the Mentalized Affectivity Scale (MAS), which I focus on in the next chapter.

The DERS is a 36-item, multidimensional self-report assessment by Gratz and Roemer (2004), which uses a 5-point Likert scale. Based on Linehan's work, the DERS highlights emotional dysregulation and has been able to predict psychopathology. The scale has six subsections: (1) nonacceptance of emotional responses; (2) difficulties engaging in goal-directed behavior; (3) impulse control difficulties; (4) lack of emotional awareness; (5) limited access to emotion regulation strategies; and 6) lack of emotional clarity. All of these subsections pull toward negative emotions. Indeed, questions 11–36 each begin with the phrase "When I'm upset . . . " Lack of awareness seems inversely related to what I have described as identifying emotions. The fact that all of the questions under the subscale for awareness of emotions are reversed might create an unintended method effect, as Lee, Witte, Bardeen, Davis, and Weathers (2016) have pointed out. Lack of emotional clarity is an important category, as it corresponds closely to what I have termed "aporetic emotions." Internal consistency of the DERS is high: alpha = .93.

A virtue of the ERQ scale by Gross and John (2003) is that, in contrast to the DERS, it looks at both adaptive and maladaptive styles of emotion regulation. The ERQ uses 10 items, examining two regulatory strategies—cognitive reappraisal (CR) and expressive suppression (ES)—through a 7-point Likert scale. Cognitive reappraisal is an antecedently focused style that is adaptive: it has consequences for affect, relationships, and well-being (p. 361). In contrast, expressive suppression uses a response-focused style that is maladaptive: it generates more negative experiences and yields a lack of authenticity. The ERQ correlates with

Big Five personality factors: CR with all but neuroticism and ES negatively with all. The ERQ seeks to measure the regulation of emotions, emphasizing control and focusing in particular, as we have seen in the discussion of the process model, on change. The average reliability for CR was alpha = .79 and for ES .73; test–retest reliability across 3 months for both scales was .69.

Hofmann and Kashdan's (2010) ASQ is a 20-item self-report measure that examines individual differences in emotion regulation. It builds on the notion that emotions can be regulated according to different styles. The authors identify three styles, extending the ERQ's distinction between cognitive reappraisal and expressive suppression by distinguishing among concealing (suppression), adjusting (cognitive reappraisal), and tolerating. Findings from the ASQ lend support to the findings from the ERQ that concealing is a maladaptive strategy for coping with negative affect. The ASQ adds an emphasis on how emotions are tolerated, particularly emotions of distress. Internal consistency was acceptable for concealing (alpha = .84), adjusting (alpha = .82), and tolerating (alpha = .68).

The ASQ seems promising, as the notion of "affective styles" suggests that personality has an impact on how someone regulates his or her emotions; however, to date, the ASQ seems to have been used less than either the DERS or the ERQ. The ASQ aspires to be theory neutral, but given what we have learned about emotion regulation in development, it remains a challenge to articulate how affective style must have its origins in attachment history. A disadvantage of all three of these measures is that the research subjects were all undergraduates and thus relatively homogeneous in age (which all of them do acknowledge as limitations). Still, they help us to understand more about normal processes of emotion regulation and provide a path to elaborate on their relation to psychopathology.

UPS AND DOWNS OF REGULATION

Let us take a closer look at how emotion regulation can be applied to psychopathology and to articulate the aim of psychotherapy. One recent estimate is that from 40 to 75% of disorders involve problems with emotions and emotion regulation (Gross & Jazaieri, 2014). In this section, I would like to zero in on difficulties with emotion regulation and reflect on their relation to specific kinds psychopathologies. I shall pursue the argument here that development is critical in terms of understanding difficulties with emotion regulation, and also address reasons to be cautious about using the term "emotion regulation." Emotion regulation has not emerged in a vacuum; it has come to the fore in a specific place and time, which valorizes individual responsibility and is skeptical of communitarianism. Personally, I am wary of the moralizing discourses that preach self-discipline, which can be associated with neoliberalism, and which obscure how dependent we are on others. Smith's memoir provides insight into the extent to which regulation depends on our relation to others (as we see in the clinical material as well). As is evident from the title of the chapter, I prefer the idea of modulating emotions, which puts the accent on experiencing and harmonizing emotions, rather than on controlling them. It is important not to obscure, though, that being unable to modulate emotions can be disastrous in social life. It can also make psychotherapy difficult: Abbass (2016) offers valuable examples of how patients' unprocessed emotions can affect therapists.

Gross and Jazaieri (2014) present an "affective science perspective" on difficulties with emotion regulation, which is based on the process model (discussed earlier). They offer a profound distinction between problems of dysregulation, or not engaging in regulation when it would be helpful to do so, and misregulation, using a form of regulation that is poorly matched to the situation (p. 389). Gross and Jazaieri make it clear that not all problems with emotions are problems of regulation. They take a significant step forward in terms of challenging the vague language of "problems with regulation" by specifying three components—intensity, duration, and frequency—and linking them to various DSM-5 psychopathologies.

Each of the three components is considered in terms of the Aristotelian extremes of too much or too little. Intensity can be seen in the hyperreactivity of social anxiety, the hyporeactivity of antisocial personality, or the hyper- and hyporeactivity of major depression. Duration can be too long, as in phobias, too short, as in PTSD, or both too long and too short, as in borderline personality disorder. Frequency can be too often, found in intermittent explosive disorder, too rare, found in dysthymia/persistent depressive disorder, or both too often and too rare, as in autism spectrum disorder. Although Gross and Jazaieri do not attempt to be comprehensive or systematic in their account, it is apparent that intensity, duration, and frequency enable them to cover a wide range of mental disorders.

In addition to delineating specific problems grappling with emotions, Gross and Jazaieri introduce the idea of emotion types, using the example of schizophrenia, to capture problems having to do with (inappropriate) behavior in context. They move on to explore how regulation (or really dysregulation) is an underlying factor in the mental disorders they are discussing. They identify three aspects of regulation: awareness, goals, and strategies. An example of hyperawareness is found in panic disorder; lack of awareness is found in eating disorders (which they discuss in relation to alexithymia). An example of dysfunctional goals, where short-term and long-term concerns are not adequately weighted, is found in bipolar I disorder. Problematic strategies can be a matter of poor choice or poor implementation: an example of the former would be found in agoraphobia, the latter in attention-deficit/hyperactivity disorder.

Gross and Jazaieri express the hope that their work might contribute to closing the gap between clinical intuition and empirical findings. Indeed, their collaboration exemplifies this aspiration, as Gross is a research-oriented social psychologist (the author of the process model and the ERQ) and Jazaieri is a cognitive-behavioral therapist trained as a marriage and family therapist, with an interest in mindfulness. They note that, ideally, emotion regulation will have to cover subclinical thresholds, not just DSM-5 categories, and that it is potentially a good fit with the Research Domain Criteria (RDoC) project, which is in pursuit of underlying mechanisms across our current diagnostic categories. The authors do not pay attention to development and thus ignore the link among attachment style, emotion regulation, and psychopathology (Abbass, 2016; Abbass & Town, 2013; Fonagy & Bateman, 2010; Fonagy, Bateman, & Luyten, 2012; Schore, 2003, 2013). Gross and Jazaieri's list of treatments that focus on emotions and emotion regulation is biased, as they completely ignore psychodynamic psychotherapy. Regardless of what one thinks of psychoanalysis, it was engaged with the concept of affect regulation long before cognitive-behavioral therapy, as behavioral therapy discounted cognition, and especially affect. The omission of psychoanalysis is curious, too, given that Gross (1998) unambiguously acknowledged psychoanalytic ideas about emotion regulation in his earlier work.

There are a number of reasons to be uncomfortable with the language of emotion regulation. It would be salutary, for example, to explore the social, cultural, and political underpinnings of emotion regulation, which certainly seem to coincide with the rise of neoliberalism. Originally, emotion regulation advocates construed the concept as closely connected to socialization and self-discipline, especially behavior that is adaptive in educational environments, thus disregarding the value of negative emotions. Moreover, there is still too little recognition of the limits on our capacity to regulate emotions and not enough consideration of the desirability of emotions being unregulated. Is there a place for unregulated emotions as distinct from dysregulated emotions? This has yet to be studied. Indeed, emotion regulation, conceived largely in terms of individual comportment, underestimates the enduring quality of co-regulation. We need to be wary about the connotations that assume voluntary conformism, which is particularly ill fitting for groups of people who have suffered discrimination and exclusion. It is neither good science nor justice if our conceptual language serves to reward the good fortune of growing up with privilege. Insofar as emotion regulation is developed as a construct, it must be distinguished from self-discipline, from good behavior that is rewarded by society and readily endorsed by mainstream social psychology.

MODULATING VIGNETTES

In this section, I offer a number of vignettes that focus on modulating emotions. What will be most striking, I suspect, is how much repetition there must be in the process of improving regulation. Underlying the notion of modulating emotions is a different perspective from models of emotion regulation that are based on a stimulus–response model. Not only does emotion regulation need to happen over time, but failure is built into the process in a sense that makes it impossible to brush aside. Clinical experience helps us to see this struggle in action, but the point is relevant to anyone—that is, not just those in therapy—who is striving to use emotions effectively.

The subject of the first vignette, Ava, is a woman in her early 40s, married with three children. She is a devoted mom and wife and runs her own successful business. She came to therapy to figure out the consequences of having been sexually abused in adolescence by a neighborhood bully, as well as being accused by her own mother of making up the abuse. In many ways, Ava had her life together and under control; yet, she was aware that there was something off about her emotions. She was bothered by how aggressively she responded to her children when they dallied in the morning before school. And she had a dim sense that she did not get upset where others might do so. In exploring her reaction to her mother's denial of her abuse, which happened contemporaneously to the abuse and again many years later when she tried to confront her, Ava claimed not to be at all angry the first time, and just a bit annoyed at the later time. It worked well in Ava's professional life to be steely and underreactive. At home, she knew that her children and husband were dismayed by her moodiness; they had to tiptoe around and not upset her.

For the first year of psychotherapy, Ava took up the process as a business plan—defining the goals and the objective means to accomplish them. Yet, she came to me knowing that I had a psychodynamic orientation and having had little success with a cognitive-behavioral therapist. I invited Ava to bring in incidents where she got angry or ones in which she thought others would think she should be angry. She did so, but in the beginning more from compliance than because she imagined this would be useful. Ava brought in examples of getting excessively angry and other examples of failing to get angry at much more important precipitants: becoming furious at her daughter who was supposed to wipe off the kitchen counter the previous evening, but not experiencing any distinct emotion after hearing that an ex-employee was cultivating one of her best clients, insisting, despite evidence to the contrary, that the ex-employee would never be successful. It would be possible to recount hundreds of incidents in which Ava was not angry, where I imagined that she would have to be angry. Thus, our work together revolved around the possibility of regulating her emotions, particularly anger, upward. As our relationship evolved, and she came to have some faith that my true motivation was to help her, she became more curious about her feelings, which meant that she could question her own reactions. Ava was able to correct the imbalance between home and work, finding more of an intermediate course, becoming less angry at home and more comfortable with being angry in social and business relationships.

In the next vignette, I return to Bernardo, whom I introduced in Chapter 1, whose dominant emotion was anger and who was able to move in the direction of feeling more varied emotions through our work together. The challenge of moving Bernardo's emotions had to do both with the misdirection of his anger (e.g., getting in an altercation at a bar after having had a fight with his girlfriend) and its disproportionate intensity (e.g., screaming at a junior coworker for ordering him a sandwich with the wrong kind of cheese). Recall from Chapter 1 that Bernardo's family suffered from excess aggression, culminating in a brutal fistfight between Bernardo and his father when he was an adolescent. So, in our work together, Bernardo had to unlearn what he learned through his early life history. He regularly failed to moderate his anger and was quite skeptical that he could ever change his behavior. However, we kept working on it, and, Bernardo started to be able to discern and track his mounting arousal, which gave him a degree of flexibility in terms of his actions.

A breakthrough occurred as Bernardo started to focus on how the consequences of his anger left him feeling unsatisfied. Some part of Bernardo never liked being part of a family culture in which the specter of violence hung over everyday life. Bernardo and I explored this history, which he had never given much thought to, and it helped him to realize that he wanted his life to be different from those of both his father and older brother. Bernardo alluded to criminal history in the family, and some of the stories Bernardo was told growing up about members of his family made them seem psychopathic. As Bernardo became more trusting of me, his hard edge softened a bit, and we were able to make some progress exploring his fears, anxieties, and fantasies. Still, we would come up against his aversion to recalling his childhood, as it was upsetting to confront. He was particularly surprised to notice a difference in how others began to perceive him. (His best friend expressed shock that Bernardo was in therapy.) Bernardo was a likable person who as a child had been expected to suppress any wish for recognition from others that was not presented in the form of a demand. When he first came to therapy, I confess that I did not expect him to stick around for long. Thus, it was a special pleasure to see that he was able to change, and to embrace a fuller, more rewarding life for himself.

In the third vignette, Charley, a man in his early 60s, came to therapy because of a history of depression but also to make sense of his life. Charley was surprisingly uninterested in change, and was resistant to my (perhaps naive) efforts to encourage him in this direction. Charley was highly intelligent and kind; he had had more success as a father (of four children) and husband (his wife was a successful banker) than at work. His father had been a hard-driving businessman who had clearly put more effort into his work than in his family. Charley's mother had been loving but anxious and had difficulty coping with life. Underlying Charley's emotional life was fear, and this fear often took on a life of its own, the way Smith's memoir suggests that individual emotions can take on the quality of fantasies. Almost everything Charley spontaneously brought up seemed to be undergirded with the anticipation of fear. Fear ranged unchecked within him; it was more than a single, discrete emotion.

It took several years of exploring how his fear was holding him back before it dawned on Charley that he could do something about it. It was almost as if he became willing to work on modulating his fear for my sake, as he was dubious of the value of such an effort. Indeed, it was only toward the end of the therapy that Charley was willing to experiment more in the present. Most of the 4 years that I saw Charley involved reflecting on his past, looking squarely at how he had missed opportunities due to his excessive fearfulness. Part of him used these explorations in order to condemn himself, and I would try to urge him in the direction of looking at himself squarely, but with more empathy. Part of him was able to reflect on himself in a way that led him to feel better about himself, although, truthfully, it could not undo what had happened in the past. Charley's desire to make sense of his life struck me as admirable, and it pushed me to reflect on my own assumptions about my role as a psychotherapist. As a therapist, it is natural to imagine that patients come in order to change, but if we tune in closely, that may not be foremost in some patient's minds. What Charley learned to do with his emotions was to own them more fully and to put fear on the back burner; as a consequence, he came to feel that he knew himself more honestly, warts and all. As I noted, Charley did become a bit more open to experimenting with change, but that was not why he sought psychotherapy and that is not what he got from it.

In the fourth vignette, Dana, a woman in her late 40s, came to therapy because she was aware that growing up in a large family, one of six siblings, was difficult and left her feeling neglected, although she was averse to connecting this early experience to any current issues in her life. Dana was a successful attorney, one of her firm's top rainmakers, but she felt she had sacrificed having a family to achieve that success. Dana was proud not to have settled for an inferior relationship. However, the quality of her actual relationships was poor, and she often ended up taking vacations by herself. Dana was self-centered, but not necessarily in a hostile or aggressive way to others. Her response to my asking her about whether she felt lonely was a terse summary comment, borrowing from the French, that she was not "dépressif." The fantasy of what her vacations would be like took precedence over her actual experience, which, I suspected, had been lonely. Her assertion of not being depressive struck me as conveying her lack of comfort with negative emotions rather than describing her inner state of mind. Dana did not have access to a wide range of emotions, and she was particularly averse to the emotion of sadness. It seemed to me that the source of her suffering was less a matter of not having the emotion than of not recognizing it or not having it available to deploy. Her defenses served to keep her from being able to use her emotions.

It took at least 3 years before Dana could accept being sad, allow herself to experience her feelings, and not attempt to minimize or cut them off. This occurred at first in fleeting moments, like when she acknowledged missing a younger colleague who had left the firm. Dana became open to less black-and-white assessments of her feelings, and more accepting of the complexity of emotions, and of the fact that they exist beyond our control. Insofar as we did talk about her childhood and early life experience, Dana described an anxious mother who verbalized her concern about her own competence and a schizoid father who spent all his free time downstairs in a workroom. Dana was an only child who became a successful student and athlete in order to gain recognition from her parents. She did not feel loved and expressed suspicion about love, as if it were relevant to other people but not to her. In her adult life, she had a series of lovers, both men and women, and had concluded that she would never be able to find the right partner. I wish I could conclude my account of Dana by offering a clear statement about the impact that therapy had on her. The best indication of change that I can assert is that I recall how terribly sad I often felt after our sessions, which became significantly less so over time. It would be hopeful to infer that the decrease in my sadness was a result of my containment of her projective identification, but it remained uncertain whether she was able to own and experience sadness.

In the fifth vignette, Edith was a young woman in her 20s whose reason for seeking psychotherapy was not apparent. She was doing well in college, had a part-time job in which she had worked her way up the ladder to have greater responsibilities, and had a few good friends from childhood. Her parents had her when they were in their mid-40s; she had a younger brother. Her family was devoutly Christian, and it was an important value for the household to remain quiet at all times. Edith was actively discouraged from becoming excited, regardless of the circumstance. For example, she recalls that after getting an A in math, which was a difficult subject for her, she gave out an involuntary shriek in telling her parents, only to be chastised by her father who was simultaneously watching a baseball game on TV.

After some time, I had the thought that one way to conceptualize Edith's problems was that joy was missing in her emotional universe. She associated joy with sin but could identify that her own values were not consistent with this assumption. I encouraged her to talk about activities that were gratifying, like listening to music. Music was a kind of private pleasure for her that she could enjoy without incurring the distress of her parents. I was wary of how psychotherapy was serving to legitimize values that were at odds with those of her family (particularly since she still lived at home). Christian rock became the embodiment of the ideal compromise formation; over time, she branched out from there into the realm of secular music.

Psychotherapy helped Edith experience pleasure as a solitary pursuit. Although she had friends, she had never had a romantic relationship. She was curious, though, and with the encouragement of one particular friend, she started to spend more time with other friends and even venture to go out to dance. She embraced dancing, it turned out, with enthusiasm and passion. Our work centered on how to preserve her connection to her family and church (the latter of which she could not imagine leaving), while allowing herself to explore the range of positive emotions. It was exquisite to witness her growing capacity to regulate her joy upwardly. This work retained some sense of danger, but we were able to ensure that her beliefs could safely remain under her control, at least in the sense that she could try to chart her own course and not capitulate to all the expectations that others had for her.

The sixth vignette concerns me, as a supervisee during my training as an intern. My supervisor was a forthright, funny psychoanalyst who identified as an interpersonalist. I liked her, but I was, from the start, uncomfortable with the direct style she used in speaking to me and recommended as a way for me to speak to my patient. It was not exactly that I disagreed with her; rather that I experienced, and I feared my patient would experience, a sense of my being on the defensive, pushed around, and led by the inclinations of another. My natural instinct was to resist my supervisor's input, and we often butted heads in our meetings. However, I didn't disagree with her suggestions about being more active in the room; it did make sense to me to try to probe my patient more than I was inclined to do.

There were times when I dreaded going to the supervision. This was less because of our butting heads (which suited both of our personalities well enough), but because I felt badly about disappointing her and perhaps inviting a negative evaluation, although I could not get myself simply to comply. In my mind, for better or worse, there was a self-image of being a virtuous supervisee or a bad-boy one. I cannot say what was in the supervisor's mind, but it certainly seemed likely in retrospect that she possessed more maturity than I had. I was surprised to observe that I was slightly amending my style in the room with my patient, as my patient was a young man who was himself reluctant to be forthcoming, and I prompted him just a bit more than I had initially done. I never uttered the sort of blunt reflections that my supervisor threw out for my consideration. I would not even say that I met her halfway. The experience in its entirety was one of appreciating that one need not be in sync with another to gain from that person's point of view. The power of this experience has grown over time.

The vignettes presented here touch on a number of aspects of modulating emotions, but like the vignettes in Chapter 1, they are in no way intended to be comprehensive. Ava modulated her emotions to be more effective—upwardly at work, where she had had trouble getting angry, and downwardly at home, where she had been overreactive. Bernardo learned to modulate his emotions downwardly—not becoming automatically enraged, not acting as soon as he was aroused—and became more adept at feeling a range of emotions. Charley became aware of fear as a central emotion and had some success in modulating it, although his achievement was more in the realm of understanding the role of fear in his life. Dana made some progress in terms of acknowledging emotions that caused her discomfort, but her difficulty owning what she felt, particularly sadness, meant that I had to be content with my own experience of feeling sad in and after our sessions, which decreased over time. Edith moved her emotions upwardly, so that she was able to seek and take pleasure in feeling joy, not just privately, but in the company of others. In the last vignette, I describe the experience of opening myself to being influenced by another, even if I did not accept the other's perspective:

the conflict between my supervisor and me helped me to heighten the emotional atmosphere with my patient in a beneficial way for me as a therapist in training and for the patient.

It is revealing that in the vignettes with Ava, Bernardo, Dana, and Edith, others figured in the process of altering how emotions were experienced and used. This supports the importance of understanding the relational quality of emotion regulation. It also provides some confirming evidence of how development has an impact on the regulation of emotions, especially insofar as this occurs along with the emerging sense of self. Admittedly, this is an early stage of articulating these ideas at this juncture in our journey. Having introduced the concept of mentalization, I explore precisely what it means to fathom emotions in light of AM in Chapters 4, 5, and 6 in Part II.

In this chapter, I have taken a step beyond identifying emotions to the processing of emotions, through the consideration of modulating emotions. I have also raised some questions about the concept of emotion regulation. As a conclusion, we could say that whereas the emotion regulation point of view affirms the Aristotelian perspective on emotions, my view preserves the tension between the Aristotelian and the Stoic perspectives. We would like to regulate our emotions, and we try to do so, sometimes successfully, sometimes not. It seems important to recognize, too, that regulation most often occurs in the context of human interaction, where both self-definition and relations to others are at stake.

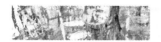 **CHAPTER 3**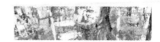

Expressing Emotions

Future research should examine whether there is a fine line
between productive inhibition of emotional expression and
counterproductive inhibition of emotional experience.
—ROLF REBER, *Critical Feeling* (2016)

In moving from identifying to modulating to expressing emotions, we
have followed a continuum of experiencing emotions in which there is
the potential for ever greater agency. However, it would be mistaken to
assume that these dimensions necessarily follow from one another. It is
conceivable that emotions can be modulated without being identified,
as I have already noted, and it is certainly possible to express emotions
without having modulated them.

What does it mean to express emotions? Darwin's book *The Expression of Emotions in Man and Animals* (1872) is the natural starting
point to engage this question: it is the source of the view that emotions
are universal and manifest in facial expressions across species. Darwin's
view has been widely adopted and developed into the so-called basic
emotions paradigm (Ekman, 1992, 2003; Ekman et al., 2003; Tomkins, 1991), which sees emotions as biological motivating mechanisms.
Interestingly, though, as Ekman (1996) observes, Darwin himself was
wary of linking the expression of emotions to communication because
he feared that this could be construed as giving credence to creationists,
even though he does make use of the idea of communication.

There is some tension between Darwin's actual views and how they
have been received. For example, Darwin (1872) differentiates between
expressions that we are aware of and others that we are not: "Screaming

or weeping begins to be voluntarily restrained at an early period of life, whereas frowning is hardly restrained at any age" (p. 222). Thus, although Darwin is typically cited as the founding figure of the paradigm of basic emotions, his belief in our capacity for emotion regulation seems qualified. Indeed, Barrett (2011), a critic of the basic emotions paradigm, argues that Darwin's actual perspective does not necessarily fit well with the basic emotions paradigm that it inspired, since he does not focus exclusively on facial emotions.

For our purposes, it is important to focus on the multiple possible meanings of expressing emotions. Facial expressions and other nonverbal behavior are part of expressions and serve to render it intelligible. However, following Barrett (2011), there is reason to question the overinterpretation of expressions as biological and universal. Evidence in support of basic emotions is slimmer than one might imagine, given how widely it has been adopted by researchers. Attempts to link basic emotions to brain function have not been successful. Moreover, recent research has challenged the recognition of basic emotions across cultures, highlighting a bias in previous research in which subjects were asked to pick from an already selected group of specific emotion categories. Expression is mediated by social construction, that is, by the particularity of the situation and its social meaning. This view is consistent with the notion of expressing emotions as a form of communication.

To what extent should we define expressing emotions in terms of verbalizing emotions? This is a hard question, especially if one wants to avoid minimizing the role of nonverbal expression. Not all cultures value verbal over nonverbal expression; to cite one example: Gendron and colleagues (2014) demonstrate that the Himba ethnic group in Namibia perceive expression in terms of physical action, rather than mental states. Thus, in placing an emphasis on verbal expression as the ideal, it behooves us to recognize that we are signaling a commitment to Western rather than universal values.

It is not surprising that the verbal expression of emotions has been critical in various measures on emotions, which attempt to look at the degree to which one can put feelings into words and communicate them to others. It is also an emphasis of most psychotherapeutic approaches to appreciate the importance of putting feelings into words as opposed to acting on them. So, we might wonder if, unwittingly, acting on emotions is demoted from being expression, or if making a distinction between healthy and unhealthy expression might be useful, as Greenberg (2015) has argued.

The etymology of "expressing" is relevant here, as it comes from the Latin, meaning to push or press out. Like the word "emotion" itself, there is movement built into the term, a trajectory outward. Revealingly, expressing seems to connote some effort or agency. In other words, an automatic outpouring of emotion might lack an aspect that determines expression. However, it would be absurd to suggest that all acting on emotions would necessarily fail to qualify as expression. The heterogeneous quality of expression is important to acknowledge (Goldie, 2000). We should also keep in mind that although there is a trajectory outward with expression, this does not negate the possibility of what I have termed the inward expression of emotions (Fonagy et al., 2002; Jurist, 2005).

Emotions are not always expressed outwardly; thus, it is crucial to my account to distinguish between their inward and outward expression. Indeed, it is the inward expression of emotions that we cultivate in psychotherapy: the value of fully experiencing emotions along with how and when they are revealed to others. Differences can exist between what is inwardly experienced and what is outwardly expressed. One might conceal one's emotions out of kindness to another or for more selfish, or even manipulative ends. Inward expression is an important and too often overlooked aspect of emotional experience; it deserves careful consideration. There is little research in this area: one recent study on smiling suggests that people suppress the outward expression of their emotions when they have outperformed others in order to accrue social benefit (Schall, Martiny, Goetz, & Hall, 2016).

Expressing emotions can legitimately be identified as the fruition of emotional experience, revealing the larger purpose of emotions as communication. Thus, we can mark a distinction between poor and good communication, recognizing the difference in quality between an emotional response that is effective in its aim and one that is not. How can we distinguish effective from ineffective emotion expression? Of course, determining "effectiveness" (or healthy versus pathological expression) would have to take up question of what is regarded as socially appropriate. There is reason to be cautious about taking normative evaluations for granted, as they might fail to take into account the intentions and self-understanding of the individual in question. (This concern will be clearer in the context of the clinical examples later in the chapter.)

One approach to understanding and evaluating the expression of emotions is developmental. Egyed, Király, and Gergely's (2013) study distinguishes between expressions that are person centered, where the caregiver is communicating something specific about what he or she feels to the infant, and those that are object centered, where the caregiver is not necessarily in the state that is being communicated but is conveying information that is generalizable and shared within the culture. As Gergely and Jacob (2012) observe, expression can aim to have an abiding, not just an episodic value. Underlying Gergely's perspective is the theory of natural pedagogy, wherein communication is used to instruct infants to become part of the culture. I say more about the communication paradigm in Chapter 4 on mentalizing emotions.

In everyday life, the expression of emotions is manifest in behavior. Outward expression can come in many different varieties: for example, it can be inhibited, it can be exaggerated, or it can seem appropriate. Insofar as outward expression often supposes another person who is receiving what is being transmitted, it can be construed in terms of inviting a response. Expressing emotions, therefore, can be integrally related to the modulation of emotions, as human beings rely on others in order to self-regulate. As noted, expressing emotions can also be unmodulated and thus undermine socially sanctioned standards.

It is important to recognize that outward expression can be indirect. Some people are more comfortable expressing emotions in mediated forms—like with music. Indirect expression can be motivated by strong feelings, so the indirectness ought not to imply diluting emotions. As Westphal, Seivert, and Bonanno (2010), have emphasized, expression ideally is flexible, adjusting itself for the specific occasion on hand. The same expression can be appropriate in one situation and not another. Flexibility is determined, in my opinion, by autobiographical history and especially by one's awareness of this history. Consider a memoir written by Ingmar Bergman, the famous Swedish film and theater director, which features complex aspects of expressing emotions.

ART AND LIFE: INGMAR BERGMAN

Ingmar Bergman's *The Magic Lantern* (1988) is a delightfully strange, frank, and revealing memoir. It is profoundly psychological in that it begins and ends with his birth and his pained relationship with his mother, grapples with his ambivalent relationship to his father, and delves into his mainly negative sibling relationships (he had a brother and a sister). On the surface, Bergman disdains and registers his discomfort with emotionality and fully recognizes the extent to which his self-centeredness has interfered with close relationships. In one sense, this memoir is not at all an obvious choice to discuss and illustrate the expression of emotions, since Bergman sees himself as rather lacking in this capacity. However, Bergman was a creative genius, one of the most profound film directors who has ever lived, and he exquisitely documents strong, subtle, multifarious emotions in his work. Bergman's films feature existential themes but also exquisitely document "the breakdown of communication between the sexes," as James Baldwin (2007) notes in his interview with the director.

Bergman's memoir begins quite literally with his birth: his mother has the flu, and the doctor delivers a gruesome verdict: "He's dying of undernourishment" (p. 1). Bergman is shipped off to his maternal grandmother and manages to survive, despite "always vomiting and . . . constant stomach-aches" (p. 1). With impish, retrospective insight, Bergman avers that "I suffered from several indefinable illnesses and could never really decide whether I wanted to live at all" (p. 1). This reflection casually overestimates his agency and at the same time hints at the self-image of being a man with a destiny.

The memoir ends with more specific information about the circumstances around the author's birth. Bergman concludes by quoting from his mother's diary: he "looks like a tiny skeleton with a big fiery red nose," he "stubbornly refuses to open his eyes," she was not able to produce milk and thus sent him away, and, rather chillingly, she considers that if he dies, she will be able to return to work (pp. 289–290). Woven into this, his mother contemplates her own mother's urging her to leave her husband (Bergman's father). The last line from the diary is auspicious: "One will probably have to manage alone as best one can" (p. 290).

Bergman moves on to describe his father and his relationship with him. His father was a parish priest whose outward demeanor contrasted with his private identity, the latter of which was "nervous, irritable and depressive" (p. 134). Bergman is devastatingly precise in capturing his father's angry outbursts over trivial matters, his oversensitivity to noise, and his overall sense of inadequacy. Bergman recalls a violent altercation between them that led him to leave home for several years. Yet, Bergman also is wary of being too hard on his father and makes room to reflect on their relationship with generosity—as on the occasion from childhood in which he almost drowns, only to have his father slap him afterward. Retrospectively, Bergman can see that his father felt guilty and remorseful for his behavior, that it was produced by fear that his son could have died, and that his father ultimately had reached out for his hand, which melted his son's rage at that moment.

The memoir depicts Bergman's family as dysfunctional and full of individual suffering. Family dynamics mix with the strict values of early-20th century Northern European Protestantism; for example, when Bergman accidentally peed in his pants, his punishment was to be forced to wear a red skirt for the rest of the day. His parents' marriage was strained by an affair his mother had, and his father's reaction of retreating into depression. Bergman did have a positive rapport with his grandmother. However, he shows little connection to his siblings. He readily confesses to having attacked his sister in her crib when she was a baby and later in life criticizes her writing, which, he avers, resulted in her abandoning it. Unsparingly, Bergman tells us that he remembers hoping his brother would die from scarlet fever, and later had a fight in which he knocked his brother's teeth out. His brother, we are informed, tried to commit suicide at one point. Bergman himself was suicidal and subsequently hospitalized as a young man.

Bergman documents his alienation and retreat from his family, and does not shy away from or distort how much that experience formed him. Bergman understands his history of anxiety as linked to his family: "my life's most faithful companion, inherited from both my mother and my father," but also "my friend spurring me on" (p. 93). He elaborates on the evolution of his own schizoid style of personality in three remarkable passages:

1. "I trusted no one, loved no one, missed no one. . . . So I was alone and raging" (p. 146).
2. "If I feel cut off, I cut off, a dubious and very Bergman-like talent" (p. 263).
3. And in the context of discussing hopeful moments of connection to others: "It is sabotaged by the peasant-like Bergman embarrassment, timidity in the face of unpredictable emotions. Best to withdraw, say nothing, evade the issue, life is risky enough as it is, thank you. Carefully, I retreat, my curiosity turned into anxiety" (p. 232).

Throughout the memoir, Bergman reveals his experience of difficulty in maintaining close relationships and his narcissistic tendencies. He is not shy about bragging that he is the world's greatest film director (p. 67). Bergman notes, "In all my misery, a well-regulated self-confidence existed, a steel column right through the ramshackle ruins of my soul" (p. 147). Yet, his narcissism has a softer edge: "I was a useless lover, an even worse dancer and a conversationalist who talked ceaselessly about himself" (p. 137). In another amusing passage, he recalls the comment of his friend, the actor Erland Josephson, that "one should be careful of getting to know people because then one started liking them" (p. 251). So, Bergman's narcissism is tempered by humor as well as by a brutal kind of self-honesty, not unlike that found in the novel *My Struggle* by fellow Scandinavian Karl Ove Knausgård (2013).[1] One of the most extraordinary examples of this brutal self-honesty is Bergman's revelation of identifying with the aggression of

---

[1] Hustvedt (2016, p. 84) quotes Knausgård from an interview in *The Observer* (March 1, 2015), saying, "I don't talk about feelings but I write a lot about feelings" (p. 84).

the Nazis as a young man and taking pleasure in giving the Heil Hitler salute during a visit to Germany in the 1930s.

Let us zero in on what Bergman has to say about expressing emotions. At first glance, what stands out is a distrust of emotions and their corresponding expression. In commenting on the fate of an older girlfriend with a passionate personality whom he learned had died at the age of 50, he observes: "That's what she got for expressing her feelings" (p. 35). He gives numerous examples of his own discomfort with emotions. Bergman dwells on his lifelong psychosomatic suffering, like his insomnia, which he compares to "flocks of black birds," and brilliantly lumps together a range of emotions: "anxiety, rage, shame, regret and boredom" (p. 63). In another description of his insomnia, he refers to the hours of 3:00–5:00 A.M. as the worst: "That is when the demons come: mortification, loathing, fear and rage" (p. 226). Bergman is more intrigued by the power of emotions than he is about the potential for emotion regulation.

Bergman is quite specific about how his emotions are usually inhibited and do not easily flow into expression. Reflecting on this, he concludes, "There was a micro-second between my intuitive experience and its emotional expression" (p. 118). This is an interesting point to contemplate. Expression that is too automatically tied to experience can be excessive and backfire; yet, expression that is mediated, as Bergman describes, can interfere with honest, forthright communication. Ultimately, Bergman seems to regard emotions as mysterious, and so expression is both necessary and unpredictable. In an astute tribute to aporetic emotions, he writes, "Ghosts, demons, and other creatures with neither name nor domicile have been around me since childhood" (p. 202).

My interest in Bergman's memoir stems, in particular, from the complexity of emotional expression it demonstrates: on the one hand, his self-reported inhibition and awkwardness as a person, on the other hand, his confident genius and intense, emotionally attuned work as an artist. These two self-images are related in Bergman's mind in that his suffering is transformed through its expression in film and theater. Perhaps artistic expressiveness is a distinct category in which unbearable emotions are sublimated and become tolerable. Such a romantic notion of the artist ought not to obscure, however, how expressing emotions can be disburdening for all of us.

MEASURING THE EXPRESSION OF EMOTIONS

There are three key measures that take up the challenge of capturing the expression of emotions. The first is the Flexible Regulation of Emotional

Expression Scale (FREE), a methodologically sophisticated measure by Burton and Bonnano (2016). The authors begin by registering their discomfort with emotion regulation scales that set up an unfair contrast between cognitive reappraisal (as desirable) and expressive suppression, especially by construing the latter in terms of frequency of behavior, rather than ability. Thus, the authors draw attention to an unidentified merit of the capacity to suppress expression. However, the authors do not explore where the capacity or ability for expression comes from; nor do they pursue issues about verbal expression per se. At the heart of this measure is an appreciation for both expression and constraint, and for the notion that flexibility of expression is a buffer against stress.

The second measure I discuss is the Grille de l'Élaboration Verbale de l'Affect (GEVA), which focuses specifically on verbal elaboration as a kind of mentalization "through the linking of words and images to unprocessed affective bodily activation" (Bouchard et al., 2008; Lecours, 1995). As the authors emphasize, verbal elaboration "highlights the quality of verbal representation associated with affect and its associated power to transform experience from impulsively expressed somaticized form of affectivity with abstract (shared) meaning" (Bouchard et al., 2008, p. 60). The measure has two orthogonal dimensions of the quality of verbalization of affect: tolerance/abstraction, which has five levels, and modalities of representation, which has four levels. Verbal elaboration is valued as the ultimate form of expression in this measure—whether someone is able to label emotions accurately and in socialized, well-defined language.

The third measure is the Affect Consciousness Interview (ACI; Solbakken, Hansen, Havik, & Monsen, 2011; Solbakken, Hansen, & Monsen, 2011), which has four dimensions: awareness of emotions, tolerance of emotions, emotional expression (nonverbal), and conceptual expression (verbal). The ACI asks about 11 specific emotions, using Tomkins's, rather than Ekman's, paradigm of basic emotions. What most distinguishes this measure is the distinction between nonverbal and verbal expression. It utilizes a 9-point scale—the Affect Consciousness Scale (ACS)—for each dimension, moving from low to high—for example, for the nonverbal dimension, from disavowal or directly irrelevant expression to finely nuanced and discriminated expression; and, for the verbal dimension, from loose characterization to a high degree of differentiation of subtle, conceptual contributions.

The ACI aims to assess "affect integration"—whether someone is able to link affects to cognition, motivation, and behavior. This is an ambitious goal, which seems to have underlying assumptions about the potential for a unified sense of agency that are not spelled out or justified. Like my perspective, though, the ACI sees the purpose of expression as communication, not just the release of individual emotions.

Both the GEVA and the ACI emphasize affect tolerance—which is interesting in that "tolerance" acknowledges an aspect of expression that is often overlooked and has only recently been incorporated into the literature on emotion regulation (e.g., in Hofmann & Kashdan, 2010, discussed in Chapter 2). It is easy to appreciate the desirability of giving up emotions or trading one emotion for another; the flip side of this would have to do with sustaining the emotion in situations in which that would be warranted—like realizing that your disappointment with a friend has reoccurred, although you have made an effort to bring the concern it to your friend's attention. Tolerance is an important contribution of theories and measures that are influenced by psychoanalysis to build in the notion of bearing the weight of negative emotions. Flexibility in expression seems like a crucial idea to develop as a research topic and is especially germane to psychotherapy, as it allows patients to have differentiated responses to situations and in relationships.

EXPRESSING EMOTIONS IN PSYCHOTHERAPY

As noted, psychotherapy has deep roots in Western culture and tends to value putting experience into words over acting them out. Currently, psychotherapy is evolving in new directions, influenced by body-focused approaches as well as contemplative practices (like mindfulness). Could it be that, by placing increasing value on nonverbal aspects of expression, we have devalued verbal aspects of expression? My inclination is to question the assumption that this is a zero-sum game, envisioning the prospect of rebalancing of nonverbal and verbal expression.

Greenberg's (2015) emotion-focused therapy offers the most developed approach to working with emotions in therapy. Rather than trying to do justice to his whole approach, though, I focus on the distinction he draws between experiencing and expressing emotions. As Greenberg observes, merely expressing emotions often does not feel satisfactory; it can help, but not necessarily (p. 18). Also, he makes the key point that the experience of feelings does not culminate with expression (p. 241).

The stated aim of emotion-focused therapy is to "give words to the moment by moment process of working with emotions" (p. 7). Greenberg recognizes that some patients will have trouble accessing and conveying their emotions; thus, he persistently recommends that therapists raise the question of where patients feel the emotion in their body. Emotion-focused therapy tries to help patients trace their emotions from the nonverbal to the verbal. Various familiar techniques are introduced, like the empty chair, in which patients can practice expressing their emotions in a less risky manner than actual interactions with others.

The job of the therapist in emotion-focused therapy is as a coach: to encourage the expression of emotion in general and, more specifically, to strive for "differentiating underlying meanings and feelings and manifestation of primary emotional states" (p. 133). The therapist is supposed to model the expression of emotion for the patient's sake (p. 213). A major emphasis of emotion-focused therapy is to help patients experience "primary emotions," which often are buried beneath "secondary emotions." Primary emotions are defined as "people's core gut responses to situations. They are our first, fundamental, most immediate visceral responses, and they can be either adaptive or maladaptive" (p. 74). Secondary emotions are responses or defenses against our primary emotions and "often obscure what people are feeling deep down" (p. 76). Greenberg sees the aim of therapists' interventions as promoting "access to the new experience of adaptive emotions and to transform old maladaptive emotions" (p. 139). He regards this approach as consistent with the work of emotional intelligence.

Greenberg provides a detailed path from the challenging process of identifying emotions to expressing them, distinguishing between health and pathology. He is comfortable with the stance that the therapist knows best, although he clarifies that the therapist derives what is best based on the patient's needs. Still: there is an unexamined normativity at the center of emotion-focused therapy that is worrisome to me. Greenberg is explicit about arguing that "expression needs to fit its social context" (p. 18). What does this mean for expression that is at odds with social context?

It makes sense to claim that expression that fits social context well will be more readily accepted; nonetheless, it might be desirable to reserve room for creative expression that bucks convention. First of all, convention changes, so creative expression can serve to expand from previously unaccepted forms of expression to new, altered ones. Or creative expression might be more revolutionary: protesting against how certain forms of expression reinforce the dominance of some group over others. An excellent example of this is found in the autobiographical memoir of Mychal Denzel Smith, *Invisible Man, Got the Whole World Watching* (2016). In that book a young African American man expresses a wide range of emotions (including fear, anxiety, and sadness) but identifies, dwells, and particularly reflects on the emotion of anger, arguing for its unmodulated expression in black rage. Citing James Baldwin, Smith defends the integrity of black rage:

> [It] has not only drawn attention to injustice; it has driven people to action, sparking movements and spurring them forward. At the very least, the public expression of black rage has allowed communities

and people who have felt isolated in their own anger to know that they are not alone. Anger is what makes our struggle visible. (p. 62)

Smith goes on to maintain that black rage serves to confront the truth of racism. And he worries about the implications of black rage diminishing. Smith's point of view is an extraordinary statement of the communicative value of expression, and needs to be incorporated into our thinking about modulating and expressing emotions. As with my critique of emotion regulation in Chapter 2, Smith shows us that there is good reason to be wary of limiting expression to societal standards, or to assume these standards are universal. Hustvedt (2016) has also persuasively argued that our assumptions about expression are gendered, in particular, with expression being associated with women. Later in this chapter, I offer a clinical example in which defiance of socially sanctioned expression expands the palette of expression for the patient and for others in a way that is refreshing and rewarding.

EXPRESSING VIGNETTES

Several vignettes serve to illustrate the issues we have confronted concerning the expression of emotions: inward versus outward expression, verbal versus nonverbal expression, the relation between expression and sociality, and the relation between self and other. As an organizing approach for these clinical examples, we might categorize expressing emotions in terms of communication that is too much or too little (and ideally, just right). However, we also consider expressions of emotion that are disjunctive, where there is a mismatch between the verbal and nonverbal expression, and expressions that are deceptive, where there appears to be an effort to mislead or manipulate the other. And we return to the vexed issue of socially sanctioned versus socially taboo expression.

The vignettes that follow help us focus on how the expressions that belong to the patient are interpreted by the therapist. There is a potentially confounding factor of the therapist's own expressions (which I address). It is a crucial part of my approach to pay attention to the dynamic between the therapist's and patient's expressive styles. Indeed, there is no reason to assume therapists are fully aware of their own expressions, given the limitations that all human beings have. Still, I would not deny that others can help us understand ourselves in a way that is impossible from the inside out.

Let us also consider other parameters—like the role of the couch, which at first glance, limits the therapist's access to the facial expressions of the patient, thus reducing data that could be informative. On a deeper level, however, the couch serves to help patients detach from normative social expectations and perhaps claim a degree of freedom. Couple and family therapy provide another kind of example, where the therapist has access to patients' emotional expressions to people other than him- or herself.

A good place to begin, as I have suggested, is with expressions that seem like either too much or too little. I describe two instances that fit both of these categories. Andrew is a successful middle-aged businessman who frequently begins sessions by stating emphatically that he is overwhelmed, sinking into the expression of his feelings in an overwrought way, ever ready to shoot down any requests from me to amplify the various situations that he is describing with more detail. My efforts to understand, in fact, elicit an increase in negativity, as if there could be no point in explaining the situations further or in imagining that together we might figure out a way to help him feel better.

Andrew was a precocious only child who was both sheltered and pushed to accomplish a great deal. In general, he was able to identify his emotions, and he was also able to moderate his emotions in specific contexts. In pursuing business, he could be charming and seductive, effectively using emotions to win people over. In his personal life (and in therapy), he tended to express his emotions excessively and crudely, especially, I came to learn, when he was not sure or was confused about his feelings. So, in experiencing aporetic emotions, Andrew would turn vociferous and intimidating to others. Over time, I realized that he felt particularly exposed with others whom he imagined could discern his state of mind, which would spark the need to put them on the defensive. Our work focused on helping him appreciate that he could trust people who cared about him to respond in a way that could benefit him. This enabled him to experience more satisfaction at home with his family.

As we might expect from knowing about him from the earlier chapters, Bernardo's expressive style was explosive: if he felt anger, he needed to rid himself of that emotion. In his family of origin, the expectation was that emotions would be expressed in this way, so to Bernardo, emotions occurred in order to be discharged. This kind of expressiveness was a communicative style that was intended to dominate and silence the person to whom expression was conveyed. Bernardo got into fistfights as a young man, including with his father, and he came to therapy in connection with his treatment for drug and alcohol abuse. He had been recommended for therapy after having completed a course in "anger management." Some of our work was aimed at helping Bernardo experience gradations of anger and broaden his responses. The more I got to know him, the more I felt he needed to expand his palette of emotions as a priority, not just rein in his anger.

For the most part, Bernardo's excessive anger was directed toward his girlfriend, family members, and occasionally coworkers. He reported constant fights with a girlfriend before she bowed to the counsel of her family and moved back to the Southwest. Bernardo had a number of incidents of road rage. I was aware of carefully monitoring his states of mind, but I recall only one occasion in which he expressed direct anger to me. He had canceled a session with little notice, and I charged him for it. I could see him tensing up as we talked this over, fighting to restrain himself against his instincts. This occurred after several years of therapy. It seemed to me a measure of his growth: his inward expression was visible outwardly but did not emerge in the way it might have in the past. Our work served to foster his realization that expressing emotions excessively was like shouting, and that he might be heard better if he toned things down.

Let us turn to consider the opposite extreme regarding expression. Clair was a young, highly intelligent woman who was shy in revealing her feelings, although it was evident that she was quite capable and reflective about identifying her emotions. It was evident, for example, that she was curious to explore aspects of her emotional experience that were below the surface, and she was nondefensive in welcoming anything I had to say. I noticed, though, that it was strikingly painful for her to put her feelings out into the world. She would take in what I said slowly; after a silence, she would begin to say something and then pause, even in the middle of a sentence. It became a joke between us: when I would inquire if she imagined that I knew what she was going to say, because the truth was, I did not know. Some patients benefit from tuning in to their emotions by inwardly expressing them. Clair could do this; what was loaded for her was the outward expression of emotion. It happened more than one time after the weekend that Clair would arrive and say that she had an important insight she wanted to tell me about. My ears perked up as I prepared to listen. I could not help but feel disappointed that it took a long time for anything of substance to emerge. I wondered whether other significant people in her life had similar experiences, as she denied that she was reacting in a different way to me. Still, her father transference to me might well have been influencing her degree of comfort. In addition, Clair's strict religious background converged with her characterological introversion to make it feel difficult to express her emotions in a way that reflected her actual feelings. I would say that we were able to make some progress, at least in terms of her wanting to share things with me.

But, in all honesty, my attempts to encourage her to be more expressive ran up against her ambivalence. Clair wanted to be understood but had a competing psychic need not to take up too much space. She was a person with a strong sense of integrity; she did not want strong emotions to spill out in the room, and she could accept that this would inhibit the potential for closeness. Clair evolved from where she started, but as she declared one morning toward the end of our work, I had never seen her cry.

David was a young man who was more obsessive than compulsive. He was a slave to his anxiety about making social gaffes; his apartment was a mess—minimal furniture, but some hoarding, with piles of clothing and uneaten food. He had trouble focusing on making changes to his living situation. He was much more invested in detailing various dramas at work, where he was accepted but often ribbed in an affectionate, rather than nasty way. David's problem was that he would be become so embroiled and stuck in narration that there would be no discernable emotional expression. My efforts to prompt expression were met with a resolute sense that nothing could help. I was heard as presenting woefully inadequate solutions, rather than, as I intended, inspiring shared curiosity about assumptions built into his understanding. One day in the context of telling me about having bought an expensive sports jacket for an event, he was debating about returning it. I asked him how he felt when he tried the jacket on in front of a mirror at home. This led to a surprising revelation, as David admitted hating the way he looked, insisting that clothes always looked better on his friends. David took this experience for granted initially, although it provided a glimpse for him of his inward expression of emotions. It provided an opening, which we were able to pursue, where there was a pattern of banishing emotional expression if and when the emotions were painful to bear.

Earl presents a variation on expressing emotions; neither too much nor too little, but an apparent disjuncture between the display and the content. It was unnerving to hear Earl describe an accident his daughter had, where she fell down a flight of stairs and required numerous stiches, because the narration was unmarked by any apparent expression of emotion on his part. When probed about this, Earl would become notably uncomfortable, affirming that he had experienced emotions (in this case, distress, with an element of guilt for not preventing the accident) but was surprised at my surprise concerning his lack of outward emotional display

Earl had a schizoid character structure, which on the surface made it seem that he was underreactive, but as McWilliams (2011) notes, can also serve to conceal strong emotions. Withdrawing in order to avoid being engulfed in no way precludes an underlying wish for closeness.[2] Earl and I worked on the disparity between what he imagined he was expressing and what the likely perception by others would be. The work was supported by the fact that Earl's wife complained about his being undemonstrative and his daughter had voiced frustration that her father was not interested in playing with her, which was not, in fact, the case.

In therapy, Earl began to experiment with expressing his emotions. At times, this seemed almost comical, and we both ended up laughing at the ridiculousness of Earl forcing himself to manufacture a new style. An important piece of our work was exploring his early life history, whereas the youngest of four children, he was often taken for granted in a busy household, shuttled around without being a part of or understanding what was happening. Earl's parents were both attorneys; his father had a small private practice and was adored by his clients; his mother worked part-time, but had been a litigator. His parents' respective occupations were a clue to Earl's sense that his father was playful but not so available, and while his mother was around more, she was on the schizoid side herself. For example, Earl had a memory that seemed to reenact his daughter's accident—in his case, swerving to miss a car on his bike, crashing, and running home bleeding, only to have his mother underreact and distractedly bandage him up at home rather than go to the hospital.

Earl was a delightful patient because he came to appreciate that he would need to adjust his expression of emotions in a way that seemed a little absurd to him but that elicited better responses from others. Earl was in a creative field, and so while he was open to making concessions to social reality in his daily life, he was adamant about not becoming too conventional. This brought home to me how much the right amount of expressiveness is socially determined, yet, without some variation and innovation, the social world threatens to become predictable and boring. There is good reason to hesitate in endorsing normative expressions, as they easily enforce a kind of conformism that patients might want and need to escape.

Frances offers another kind of expression of emotions. She was a woman in her late 50s, an unhappy veteran of the mental health care

---

[2]Schizoid phenomena are complicated for numerous reasons. First, they span the range from serious psychopathology to people who have to be considered fairly healthy. Second, they lie at one end of a continuum that has at the other end relatedness, yet this does not overlap with a distinction between sickness and health. Third, in my experience, there are some schizoid people who crave closeness with others (as I am suggesting with the patient in question above), but some who really want and need distance between themselves and others.

system, whose serious psychopathology (bipolar disorder and a personality disorder) was buried under a wealth of complaints, suggesting that her doctors had made her ill. Frances was a difficult patient to work with because moments of connection had to be immediately undermined; so, progress in therapy was often followed with a fresh outpouring of negativity. Although this was not easy to endure, at least the emotions in the room were authentically felt. One of the most disturbing aspects of working with Frances was, as it eventually dawned on me, her persistent deceptive self-expression. Some of this false expression was unintentional, and though it was confusing, it did not deflect my empathy for her. Some of the false expression was intentional, which was harder to accept. It was uncomfortable to realize Frances's interest in deceiving me about her past and her efforts to influence, manipulate, and control others.

It did not seem productive to encourage Frances to explore her family history or her history in various institutions and therapies. Along with the multiple diagnostic labels that she had received, it was evident that she had suffered from a history of complex trauma. She had crafted answers to historical questions, so my work moved to focus on her feelings in the present and her reactions to me. Still, we were operating with different assumptions: mine was that her expression of emotions would help me understand her better; hers was that she would use it to induce a kind of learned helplessness and defeat by deceptively shifting gears, rather than divulging her real feelings. It was as if her ability to communicate had been co-opted by a system that instrumentally sought to prevail over or escape from me, away from any hint of connection.

Was I able to help Frances at all in therapy? There were moments in which I would have answered affirmatively: the fact that she often expressed hatred toward me did not mean that she really felt that way or even that she did not find me likable enough. In the long run, our work was aborted when Frances spontaneously acted on a desire to move to another city. She had brought this idea up many times, and we had assessed the choice as questionable, given that she had no place to live, no job, and no friends or support system. Off she went; but she came back after a few months and returned to therapy. During the second course, Frances was angrier, and her anger spread to anyone she encountered, including me. She quit therapy, gleeful that she had vanquished me. Even now, she will occasionally call me up, leaving rambling, accusatory messages. When I have responded, it seems to make her more upset. I do not believe it was impossible to treat such a disturbed patient, but I make no claim to having opened her to a more rewarding way of communicating emotions.

Gayle was a transgender patient who was transitioning from male to female. She had a genetic disorder with mixed anatomy and had a powerful, lifelong transference to the institution in which I was seeing her. As a 6' 3" woman, Gayle garnered unwanted attention and stares while riding the subway. She hated being stared at and had interesting ways of dealing with it, like arriving at a session and immediately trying to put me on the defensive by commenting on what I was wearing. She herself dressed flamboyantly, which of course produced a predictable initial reaction on my part of worrying that how she might be seeking out some of the negative attention she received. Our work centered on her right to self-expression: although she had always felt like a woman, this did not mean that she would not have to practice being a woman in public. Ironically, when we think of expressing emotions authentically, we tend to assume that it goes hand in hand with unique individuality. In the case of Gayle, she self-consciously sought to work on her self-presentation as a woman. This meant helping her choose to wear high heels, although this elevated her height to 6' 6" or so. While conventional wisdom might have pushed us in the direction of helping her to fit in, allowing her the space to make the choice to fit while standing out was effective.

Let me conclude with another example from a case that Leary (2012) reports. Her patient was an African American man in his 20s who was an overachiever, having gone to the right schools and landed a plum job at a consulting firm. On this job, the patient, who is referred to as Dean, runs into trouble as he senses his exclusion from invitations extended to others by his boss, who graduated from the same college as Dean. Leary traces Dean's understandable anger and frustration to having grown up with an infirm father who passed away. Yet, Leary is also not satisfied by formulating a psychodynamic hypothesis. Racism, as she observes, embodies the opposite qualities of both being hyperreal and a fantasy. The case is fascinating, as it documents how emotional expression is governed by the perception of others. When Dean runs into trouble at work, he will suffer the consequences as a rare model-minority employee. Through therapy, Dean is able to channel his understanding of implicit racism productively, which results in his getting back on track.

The patients Earl, Gayle, and Dean challenge universal assumptions about the expression of emotions. People who belong to the dominant culture have more latitude when it comes to the expression of emotions and are less vulnerable to suffering the consequences of being too visible. Thus, when we conceptualize expression in terms of too much or too little, we cannot afford to forget to ask, "For whom?" All cultures apply pressure for people to conform; the pressure is escalated when it comes to people who deviate from the norm.

All therapists—regardless of their orientation—have an obligation to take into account their own social position as part of how they understand the patients with whom they work. Although psychodynamic psychotherapy already has the concept of countertransference, it is important not to minimize the impact of specific, concrete aspects of identity (like race, gender, and social class).

COMMUNICATING EMOTIONS

The study of emotions through facial expressions is venerable and remains a vital focus of research on emotions, however controversial it might be. My frame has been wider: to conceptualize expression in terms of communication. Perhaps, the most important point that has emerged is that there is an implied other in the expression of emotions, even if we concede that it is possible for someone to be crying or fuming while sitting alone in a room.

Communicating emotions typically involves a sender, a receiver, and a message. It can be viewed from an interpersonal perspective, as with the cases that have been discussed. Nonverbal expressions, like facial expressions, can be informative, but verbal expression has a special importance culturally, and especially for the enterprise of psychotherapy. As I have argued, expression can be inward or outward. Psychotherapy can be understood as an experimental lab in which emotions are practiced—in session, one can express emotions freely, regardless of whether one will then express them outside. It bears emphasizing that outward expression is not always desirable; inward expression can be part of an effort to engage in more sensitive communication, and so knowing when to express emotions inwardly or outwardly is a crucial skill to develop in psychotherapy (more on this in Chapters 6 and 7).

Even in the case of Bergman's autobiographical narrative, where he confesses the desire to keep others at a distance, on a more subtle level the need for others is acknowledged. Moreover, as a brilliant artist, Bergman is a special example whose messy life is distinct from the depth of emotion that is portrayed in his films.

The clinical vignettes also support the interpersonal component of the expression of emotions—though of course the aim of communication is not met in all of these cases. The case examples highlight, first, the contrast between a style of expression that is excessive (Andrew and Bernardo) and one that is deficient (Clair and David). I then move on to add other variations: Earl, where there is a disjuncture between what is expressed and what is felt, and Frances, where there is deception between what is expressed and what is felt. In addition, my vignettes included examples (Gayle and Dean) that push us to recognize that expression is mediated by social and cultural factors, and thus we should refrain from blithely assuming that it must be the same for everyone.

Indeed, expression as communication is socially embedded. While expression has a cathartic element, as psychoanalysts first articulated, it serves other purposes, too. In fact, Freud moved beyond thinking of affects as discharge phenomena when he recognized "signal affects," which convey meaning. Expression is more than simply the release of energy. Expressing emotions is a way to convey meaning, and that meaning is established and maintained as social order. Some, like Greenberg, see their role as therapists or coaches to help clients adhere to the social order. I am wary of this, both because I am averse to endorsing the social order automatically, and because I have a strong investment in avoiding imposition on my patients.

Expressing emotions has an interpersonal aspect, a social aspect, but it also can be mediated by creative self-expression, which has the potential to alter interpersonal and social relationships. Not everyone can be Bergman, but we all can work on our ability to express emotions better and thus communicate more successfully. In later chapters, I describe what this looks like.

As discussed in Chapter 2, the Aristotelians are optimistic about our potential to educate our emotions and their expression; Stoics are more skeptical, although at least some philosophers, like Spinoza, put the emphasis on waiting until the power of the emotion subsides, that is, delaying the expression of the emotion until it is fully experienced. From a clinical standpoint, one would wonder whether some patients fall into the Aristotelian category and others into the Stoic category, just as some patients with addiction issues can embrace moderation and others cannot.

If psychotherapy is effective, it will have implications for how patients express their emotions. The ultimate test of this is shepherding patients to express their emotions in their lives, outside of the sheltered space of the consulting room. This can be a challenging goal that takes practice and effort no matter what skills one possesses naturally. Therapy is a social institution that exists on the boundary of the social order, not fully out and not fully in, which allows for a unique opportunity to foster the advancement of communication. The purpose of therapy is to benefit individuals' lives, but it would be a mistake to ignore its larger social implications.

Coda

Before delving into my approach to clinical practice, I would like to address the relation among the three elements of emotional experience: identifying, modulating, and expressing emotions. As we have seen depicted in the illustrative cases so far, people can have problems with each of these elements (and, of course, with combinations of them or all of them). Clarifying and assessing where patients' problems are is a first step toward being able to help them.

Preliminary evidence from my research suggests that these three categories fit well with how subjects think about different components of their emotional experience (see the discussion of measuring mentalized affectivity in Chapter 4 and the Mentalized Affectivity Scale in the Appendix). These three elements are related to one another, and they overlap in function. As we have already noted, an interest in identifying emotions can shade into trying to adjust them, and the effort to modulate emotions can have an impact on how they are expressed.

Identifying, modulating, and expressing emotions often form a sequence in which we become aware of, experience, and act on our feelings. A sense of agency is a part of each of these elements; however, as I mentioned earlier, there is a movement in the direction of greater agency in the path from identifying to modulating to expressing emotions. Identifying emotions indicates the inception of agency; modulating the actualization of agency; and expressing the realization of agency.[1]

---

[1] On the theme of agency from philosophical perspectives, see my book *Beyond Hegel and Nietzsche* (Jurist, 2000).

Most people have some awareness of their emotions and are responsive when they are encouraged to be curious and explore their feelings further. Insofar as that curiosity is rewarding, their curiosity will increase. Yet, it cannot be denied that some people are not aware of their emotions and thus are likely to lack curiosity. Often people seek out psychotherapy because they have some awareness of their emotions, but that awareness is mixed with defensiveness or distortions. People with alexithymia are unaware of their emotions to a surprising degree. They do not seem to feel what we imagine one would feel in specific situations, and it is difficult to engage them to be more curious. At the other extreme, it is possible for a person to exhibit a false confidence about his or her emotions, mistaking them or using them in an idiosyncratic way. Curiosity will not be easy to inspire in such a person. And indeed all of us have ways of avoiding painful emotions. Thus, it is a part of therapies of every orientation to encourage honest experiencing of emotions.

Practice is required to improve one's skill in identifying, modulating, and expressing emotions. Identifying emotions will include naming them, but also expanding the range of emotions one is aware of and being comfortable with uncertainty. Modulating will include adjusting and refining emotions, but also an appreciation of the relational context that in most cases stimulates the process. Expressing emotions concerns making the emotions manifest in the world, but more perspicuously, being able to know when to manifest them outwardly or inwardly. Expressing emotions reminds us that emotions do not exist apart from sociality, which does not mean that they cannot be at odds with the values of a particular culture.

Having assessed where a patient needs the most help, the therapist's job is to focus on building the patient's skills in that area. It would be unusual for a patient not to benefit from help in all areas, so I would encourage a therapist to prioritize, but not to focus on just one area at the expense of others. A good entry point is where the therapist can gain some traction in terms of inspiring the patient to be curious about his or her emotions. However, we should keep in mind that although curiosity is a helpful predictor of the length and difficulty of the road that lies ahead, it must be developed further in ways that I describe in Part II. Curiosity, we can conclude, is a necessary but insufficient condition for experiencing emotions fully.

The autobiographical writings that I cite supplement the clinical material. The memoirs depict a person in context, so emotions are embedded in the narrative, and there is freedom from the pressure to tell a story of things being bad and then getting better. Certainly, the narratives have an investment in depicting learning and growing. As a creative pursuit, however, writing is used to fathom and convey the authors' experience. It is possible to see the choice to write an autobiographical memoir as an expressive, therapeutic activity. Indeed, it would be fascinating to ask these authors to compare themselves before and after their projects.

The memoirs I have used do not fit neatly into the elements of identifying, modulating, and expressing emotions. As expected with a comedian, Sarah Silverman zooms from the profound to the silly and back again. Her depiction of fear, augmented by several traumatic events, is not simply about a single, discrete emotion. Silverman links her fear to her motivation to perform onstage, using the emotion to overcome herself, although it is not thereby eradicated. The notion that an emotion that holds us back but still exists in the background can be transcended is an illuminating point that, to my knowledge, has not been researched.

Silverman's memoir is compulsively self-revealing, both affirming and deftly parodying a bathetic style of autobiographical writing. She plays at being narcissistic, but she offers hope to readers who have suffered from fear, anxiety, depression, or enuresis and who have sought psychotherapy for help. Furthermore, Silverman's narrative touches on her efforts to modulate her emotions and also express them. As a Jewish woman from New Hampshire, Silverman's identity is based on being an outsider. As a comedian in the spirit of provocateurs like Lenny Bruce, Silverman enjoys expressing herself in shocking ways—discussing scatological topics explicitly as a way to challenge norms of conventional discourse.[2] Her autobiographical memoir is a study of someone who knows who she is and what she believes, and who takes pleasure in making us laugh and think at the same time.

The memoir by Tracy Smith, whose mother died when she was 22 years old, is her effort to work through her grief. The writing is restrained compared to Silverman's, which is appropriate to her focus on mourning. The story captures the close relationship between mother and daughter and the extent to which Smith's effort to establish her own identity occurs in relation to her mother. Smith weaves a complex narrative, though, as she feels the pull both toward and away from her mother. My focus is on her experience of modulating the experience of mourning and loss. However, Smith conveys a wider assortment of emotions along the way, including guilt (for seeking her own independence away from her mother) and fear (questioning how she will find her way apart from her family).

---

[2] Alice Gregory (2015), writing in the *New York Times,* reflects on how comedians have assumed the role in our society once held by social critics, specifically mentioning Sarah Silverman.

Smith defines herself through defining her relationship to her mother. She shows us a path young adults can use to distinguish themselves from their parents (manifested through her questioning of religion), yet to affirm new ways of remaining connected to them (her writing exemplifies this). Currently 45 years old and director of the creative writing program at Princeton University, Smith has had great success as a writer—a book of her poems won a Pulitzer Prize in 2012 (Smith, 2011), her memoir *Ordinary Light* was nominated for a National Book Award in 2015, and she was named poet laureate of the United States in 2017. Smith strongly identifies as a poet and joked in a reading of her memoir at Labyrinth Books in Princeton, New Jersey, on April 1, 2015, that for her prose was a "foreign language." As an African American, Smith proudly defines herself in the lineage of her mother, who was involved in the civil rights movement, even if she wrestles with ambivalence toward her mother's religious commitments.

In discussing the memoir of Ingmar Bergman, I focused on his struggle to express his emotions. Like other well-known artists—Picasso comes to mind—there is a strong contrast between the ruthlessness and messiness of the life and the exquisite beauty and profundity of the creative work. Bergman was egotistical, but he was also, without question, a brilliant filmmaker. Although I do not discuss his films, they are remarkable for providing glimpses into the interior lives of the characters and their relationships. The camera moves closer in painful scenes rather than distancing itself, as the viewer might expect. The emotional honesty depicted in Bergman's films is intense, and helps us realize that we can bear suffering.

Bergman is quite articulate about his difficulties with emotions, that is, with identifying, and especially with modulating them. He is candid and open about his frequent experience of aporetic emotions. Bergman's personal struggles are faced forthrightly and dealt with psychologically, insofar as they are traced back to his relationship to his mother, by whom he felt abandoned, the tense explosiveness of his family life, and the struggle to fit within a strict Scandinavian ethos. Bergman epitomizes the spirit of the kind of autobiographical memoir in which it is self-defeating to make oneself look better than one is. Bergman is not so likable in the memoir, but I do not know of any autobiographical writing that exceeds it in prizing truthfulness over everything else.

Throughout Part I, I have examined aspects of emotional experience, paying attention to where someone might have strengths or difficulties. In Part II we engage the question of how AM has an impact on the experience of emotions. We take a step beyond how one actually handles emotions to consider how one might ideally do so.

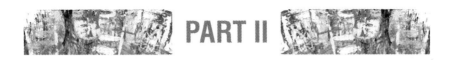

PART II

MENTALIZED AFFECTIVITY

We may mentalize a great deal, but that doesn't mean we
always do it well or that we can't do it better.
                        —MATTHEW D. LIEBERMAN, *Social* (2013)

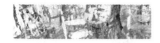 CHAPTER 4

Mentalizing Emotions

We cannot have a credible theory of mind without a
credible understanding of the basic emotional feelings we
inherit as evolutionary tools for living.
—JAAK PANKSEPP AND LUCY BIVEN,
The Archaeology of Mind (2012)

As I argued at the end of Part I, it is important for therapists to clarify
where patients need help with emotions and to focus attention on those
specific areas. However, our job is not merely to help patients to locate
where they live but to inspire them to undertake new ventures. Part II
takes on the challenge of helping people improve their understanding
and experience of emotions through mentalizing them. This chapter will
require a bit of a detour, as I begin by explicating the concept of mentalization—exploring where it comes from, how it pertains to psychotherapy, and how it has been measured. In this chapter, I also introduce the
concept of mentalized affectivity, which I have been writing about over
the last decade and a half (Fonagy et al., 2002; Jurist, 2005, 2008, 2010,
2014), and which will be amplified over the subsequent three chapters.
Mentalized affectivity is the process of making sense of emotions in light
of one's autobiographical memory (AM) and history. The concept is akin
to emotion regulation, but it is rooted in context and sense of self. Mentalized affectivity includes identifying, modulating, and expressing emotions, but it is something more: the fruition of what psychotherapy can
accomplish.

This chapter tilts in a theoretical direction, and readers who prefer
to remain on the main highway are welcome to skip the opening section,

as it navigates intellectual sources and debates about mentalization before shifting to the topic of mentalizing emotions in psychotherapy. I show how Fonagy and colleagues have adapted mentalization theory and raise questions about the applicability of mentalization in psychotherapy, and then turn my attention to mentalized affectivity. This chapter culminates with a description of various measures of mentalization as well as the measure of mentalized affectivity that my research team has created. (See the Appendix for the Mentalized Affectivity Scale.)

The clinical ramifications of mentalized affectivity are drawn out in subsequent chapters. In Chapter 5, I move on to address the clinical assessment of mentalized affectivity, incorporating research about AM, returning to autobiographical narrative (the case of Oliver Sacks), and discussing clinical material about improving mentalized affectivity. In Chapter 6, I elaborate on the idea of mentalized affectivity as therapeutic action, placing it in the context of the communication paradigm and the enterprise of psychotherapy itself. In Chapter 7, I examine mentalized affectivity in relation to other contemporary psychoanalytic theories. In the Conclusion, I voice an argument for a more interdisciplinary approach to psychotherapy, which my book has sought to exemplify.

SOURCES OF MENTALIZATION

Interest in the concept of mentalization is increasing significantly, as the chart in Figure 4.1 indicates.

Yet, mentalization continues to have an uncanny aura in the sense that it seems both familiar and strange, and readily comes in and out of focus. Numerous questions remain about its meaning, especially concerning its relevance in the field of clinical psychology.

A fundamental concern in this chapter will be to convey the importance of the construct of mentalization, which has been brought into psychotherapy through the work of Peter Fonagy and colleagues. However, in order to make sense of the construct and to enumerate its various connotations, I begin by providing a kind of genealogy of where the term comes from. Not only will this give the reader a deeper appreciation of the meaning of the concept, it will help us to explore its evolution and its future development.

THE FRENCH PSYCHOSOMATIC VIEW OF MENTALIZATION

There are two main sources for the idea of mentalization, which can be defined as the capacity to understand and interpret behavior in terms of

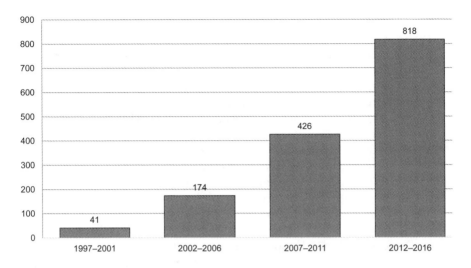

FIGURE 4.1. Proliferating references to mentalization in PsycINFO (1997–2016).

mental states, whether our own or others. The objects of mentalization are broadly construed: ideas, beliefs, and values, as well as emotions. "Mentalization" is a widely used term in cognitive science, incorporating long-standing philosophical problems from "philosophy of mind" and newer, cross-disciplinary problems from "theory of mind." However, it is less well known that the term "mentalization" was first used by French *psychosomaticiens* like Pierre Marty, who used the term in the 1950s as a way to challenge mind–body dualism and to affirm that having a mind depends on reading one's own bodily states.

The French school of psychosomatics is closely tied to psychoanalysis. A premise of this perspective, which focuses on how we understand our own minds, dwells upon the reciprocal interaction with our bodies. It is mistaken in their view, for example, to mark a distinction between mental and physical disorders, given that all physical disorders necessarily have mental aspects. Marty worked as a hospital psychiatrist, putting his ideas to use in treating patients with cancer and other serious illnesses. In encouraging mentalizing with such patients, Marty and Leighton (2010) offers a broad point of view that seeks to link the physiological with the social though the psychic.

This approach to psychosomatics has more in common with the still-surviving German perspective on psychosomatics—best symbolized by von Weizsäcker, who held a broad view of psychosomatics as "the introduction of the subject in medicine" (Frommer, 2013; Greco,

1998)—than it does with the now antiquated approach of Alexander (1950), which posited that specific physical disorders were caused by specific emotional problems. Currently, excitement about the progress of neuroscience has diminished interest in psychosomatics; however, there is a kind of revival of psychosomatics that has resurfaced through mind–body research (Gottlieb, 2013; Gubb, 2013).

The French psychosomatic perspective tends to affirm mentalization in relation to its failure. Marty was fascinated by patients who "dementalize" or fail to mentalize, which he links to *"pensée opératoire,"* a kind of concrete thinking devoid of fantasy and/or recalled dreams and in which little symbolic activity exists. Aisenstein (2006), a second-generation member of the French psychosomatic school, stresses the link between operational thinking and trauma. Bouchard and Lecours (2008) provide an illuminating gloss on how to define and spot operative thinking: tangential associations, words that reduplicate action, stereotyped expressions, clichés, and conformism, thoughts and memories that are not related in a coherent framework, not using context to create meaning, and an empty presence (or "white relationship") that lacks reference to an inner, live object or self (pp. 110–111)[1]. Marty (Marty & M'Uzan, 1963) observes that patients like this present as if everything happens to or is imposed on them (p. 348). In this account, mentalizing entails the capacity for psychic representation but necessarily relies on the effort to read and make sense of bodily experience.[2] It is closely tied to the Freudian paradigm that thinking grows out of frustrated wishes. The consequences of not mentalizing are serious, and can be fatal. We need to mentalize as a hedge against the domination of our own powerful affects and drives.

THE COGNITIVE SCIENCE VIEW OF MENTALIZATION

The cognitive science perspective emphasizes how we understand, or "read," others' minds—a profound departure from the psychosomatic perspective. Two alternative, and seemingly opposed, points of view have been put forth to explain mentalization: theory theory and simulation theory (Baron-Cohen, Tager-Flusberg, & Cohen, 2000; Carruthers & Smith, 1996). According to the former, the capacity to interpret the

---

[1]The idea of a "white relationship" corresponds to what we might think of as a bland relationship or a tepid transference, where affective connection appears to be weak, undeveloped, and unrecognized.

[2]Green (2010) observes that Marty never defined exactly what he means by representation.

mind of another is based on formulating a theory of how minds work, which corresponds to our shared beliefs or "folk psychology."[3] According to simulationists, the capacity to interpret the mind of another is predicated on placing oneself in the other person's situation. Simulationists argue that we extrapolate from ourselves in reading others. Mentalization, by this account, relies on our ability to go "offline" and put ourselves in the "mental shoes" of others, as Goldman (2006) avers. Gordon (1996) observes that simulation is a matter of imagination and the suspension of our own reactions. Gordon also observes that the virtue of the simulationist view is that it is based on "hot cognition," which includes emotions, rather than the "cold cognition," which theory theory seems to presume.

An issue worth noting is that the theory-theory position was based on so-called "false-beliefs" experiments that use switched-location tasks to suggest that mentalization emerges around 3–4 years old, as children younger than that struggle to recognize that others might *not* know what they know—that is, that others might hold a false belief based on having limited knowledge compared to the child's own knowledge.[4] New research complicates this picture by demonstrating earlier mentalizing abilities: already at 15 months old, infants monitor other agents and infer, attribute, and represent the beliefs of others (Onishi & Baillargeon, 2005). Indeed, there is research suggesting that infants as young as 7 months are able to read the minds of others in a rudimentary way (Kovács, Teglas, & Endress, 2010). Of course, evidence in support of early mentalization does not necessarily rule out an important shift taking place at 3–4 years old (see Ensink & Mayes, 2010; Gergely & Jacob, 2012). It does certainly raise the point that mentalization ought to be conceived of dimensionally and as an ongoing process.

---

[3] Some theory-theory proponents are infatuated with the analogy between the trial-and-error process of children and what scientists do (Gopnik 1993; Gopnik, Capps, & Meltzoff, 2000). This idea is controversial, however, and has been criticized as being misleading and not well developed (Bogdan, 1997; Goldman, 2006). Recently, Legare and Harris (2016) have made the intriguing proposal that the child is like an anthropologist, charged with discerning and integrating emotional and cultural learning.

[4] As Carruthers and Smith (1996) describe it, "The original false-belief task involved a character, Maxi, who places some chocolate in a particular location and then leaves the room; in his absence the chocolate is then moved to another location. The child is then asked where Maxi will look for the chocolate on his return. In order to succeed in this task, the child must understand that Maxi still *thinks* that the chocolate is where he left it—the child must understand that Maxi has a false belief, in fact" (p. 2).

There have been some recent efforts to move the cognitive science perspective on mentalization beyond the either/or quality of the original debate. Given what he sees as the shortcomings of both the theory-theory and simulation approaches, for example, Gallagher (2011) proposes a new perspective, which he labels the "interaction theory." It begins from the premise that others are not as mysterious as either theory theory or simulation theory suppose. According to Gallagher, we have intuitive, immediate ways of interacting with others that might not count as actual mentalizing but that contribute to social cognition. Apperly and Butterfill (2009) introduce a two-track system of mind reading: an early version that is efficient but inflexible and a more complex version that helps us account for mind-reading abilities such as the ability to discern false beliefs. Their perspective, which derives from number cognition, is mainly focused on reasoning about beliefs, rather than processing emotions.

Recent hybrid accounts represent the effort to incorporate both theory theory and simulationism.[5] Goldman (2006) offers a compelling example, which is mainly a defense of simulation theory but makes some room for theory theory. Goldman proposes that simulation relies upon "pretense," an act of imagination in which we aspire to make sense of what others might be experiencing and then to attribute beliefs to them. Yet, Goldman (Shanton & Goldman, 2010) concedes that some mind-reading predictions do not exclusively rely on simulation, but benefit from incorporating theory (p. 174).

Goldman (2006) emphasizes that simulation requires us to quarantine our own beliefs for the sake of understanding someone else. The metaphor of quarantining is meant to convey the importance of keeping one's own beliefs separate and the danger of allowing egocentrism to interfere with our judgment. Mistakes occur, in this account, because of a failure to bracket one's own real point of view (p. 148). Goldman suggests that "egocentric biases" can explain why such failures occur, but he ultimately registers faith in our ability to discern introspectively the boundaries between self and other.

Goldman's theory is intriguing because it highlights various dimensions of mentalization and marks the complexity of the idea. His

---

[5] Wilkinson and Ball (2012) and Mitchell, Currie, and Ziegler (2009) argue that we should strive to move beyond viewing the two perspectives as opposing each other and seek to combine them. Bach (2011) defends a version of the hybrid account that accentuates their interrelation, based on the theory of structure mapping.

[6] Lombardo, Chakrabarti, and Baron-Cohen (2009) and Heyes and Frith (2014) have also argued in favor of distinguishing between two levels of mentalization: low-level embodied/simulative representations and high-level inferences.

distinction between "low" and "high" mentalization is critical (the full implications of which will be discussed later).[6] Briefly, low mentalization typically concerns detecting emotions, especially facial expressions, and pains. It is relatively simple, primitive, automatic, and largely below consciousness (Goldman, 2006, p. 113). High mentalization involves mental states that are relatively complex, subject to voluntary control, and have some degree of accessibility to consciousness (p. 147). It typically involves "propositional attitudes," units of thought that purport to be true or false (Shanton & Goldman, 2010). Most importantly, the high level of mentalization requires the use of pretense or enactment imagination—that is, it is not mere abstract conjuring, but a willingness to experiment with the beliefs. Goldman specifically connects high mentalization to self-reflection or self-reference, the ability to engage in self-investigation in the context of third-person mentalizing. High mentalization can be distinguished from low mentalization because it is likely to be more precise and accurate.[7]

To summarize: Low mentalization concerns emotions; high mentalization concerns emotions as well but is conditioned by the capacity to regulate and modify them. According to Goldman, high mentalization depends on imagination, a specialized function that allows us to grapple with the complexity of social life. Thus, mentalization is less an online function governing competitive situations in which we need to know how to act than it is a function that reflects our having an interior life that is defined by its search for understanding. Emotions are just as important in high mentalization, but they are harnessed to context and meaning. It is this level of mentalization that is particularly relevant for psychotherapy.

USING MENTALIZATION IN PSYCHOTHERAPY

There is clearly a vast contrast between the perspectives of the French psychosomatic school and cognitive science on mentalization. The French psychosomatic perspective sees mentalization in terms of affects, drives, and the body. The cognitive psychology perspective is freighted

---

[7]Another philosopher, Stueber (2006), has proposed a distinction between basic and reenactive empathy that closely resembles the distinction that Goldman makes between low and high mentalization. In the context of defending simulation theory, Stueber contrasts "basic empathy," which he sees as a fundamental perceptual level of interpersonal relations, and "reenactive empathy," which requires a richer awareness of context and meaning. Reenactive empathy leads us not just to identify what is going on with another person, but to seek to make it intelligible.

toward cognition. Moreover, the main focus of the French psychosomatic perspective on mentalization is that it concerns one's relation to
oneself, whereas the cognitive psychology perspective is that it mainly
concerns one's relations to others. The French psychosomatic perspective construes mentalization in the interstices of body and mind, as
opaque and inscrutable, whereas the cognitive science perspective tends
to see mentalization more straightforwardly, presuming that it works
effectively, with some qualification (Nichols & Stich, 2003).

Indeed, the question arises whether these two perspectives are
dealing with two fundamentally different constructs, although the
same term is used. Fonagy has developed an ambitious framework that
aspires to encompass and integrate all of the perspectives we have discussed. Instead of pitting affects versus cognition, mentalization theory
affirms the value of both with the concept of mentalized affectivity, as
will become apparent. Instead of seeing the mind as opaque or transparent, mentalization acknowledges the struggle to find granularity. Instead
of dwelling on the other or the self, mentalization theory offers a new
perspective in which both are appreciated. Mentalization evolves from
primary caregivers' (others') mentalizing about the self to the self being
able to mentalize about itself.

Although mentalization is a unique idea, it also bears the legacy of
previous psychoanalytic theory: from ego psychology, the self-observing
ego, object relations, Winnicott's holding environment, and Bion's containment (Steele & Steele, 2008). A virtue of the mentalization construct
is that it has less metapsychological baggage than previous psychoanalytic accounts and is more receptive to sources outside of psychoanalysis.
I return to the relation between mentalization and related constructs in
the next section (and again in Chapter 7).

It should be noted that Fonagy and colleagues' (2002) understanding of mentalization has evolved from the idea that mentalization is a
developmental skill that grows out of (ideally secure) attachment, good-
enough caregiving, and the nurturing of the emergent self. This idea was
amended for several reasons. First, as argued by Gergely and Unoka
(2008) and discussed above, mentalization has an earlier origin than 3–4
years old, which the false belief paradigm assumed, and seems to have
its own trajectory distinct from attachment. Second, greater subtlety has
emerged in our understanding of borderline personality disorder: that it
was less the case that borderline patients could not mentalize than that
their capacity to mentalize diminished in circumstances in which their
arousal level resulted in the activation of their attachment systems. It is
important, therefore, to appreciate that attachment and mentalization
actually can function antagonistically (Fonagy & Target, 2008). Third,
as the concept of mentalization has developed, flawed variations have

been identified, such as hypermentalization and hypomentalization, rendering it more complex. Fourth, there is now a much greater appreciation of the fact that mentalization is context driven (we behave differently in different settings) and can vary depending on relationships (Bateman & Fonagy, 2015). Finally, there is movement toward accommodating a communication paradigm rooted in human evolution, in which mentalization is specifically tied to the capacity for epistemic trust (see Fonagy & Campbell, 2015; Fonagy, Luyten, & Allison, 2015).

Recent scholarship (Bateman & Fonagy, 2012; Luyten & Fonagy, 2015) delineates four distinct aspects of mentalization: automatic and controlled, internal and external focus, self and other, and cognitive and affective. One needs flexibility and balance in order to negotiate these four polarities. The distinction between automatic and controlled contrasts implicit, everyday interactions and explicit processes that rely on inhibition of neural systems, and it seems related to the distinction Goldman and Stueber make between low and high mentalization.

It would seem psychotherapy would aim to improve high mentalization, although it is an empirical question whether low mentalization can be modified (and how this might affect the high level). It remains unclear whether the two levels are categorically different, or whether high mentalization grows out of low mentalization. Lombardo and colleagues (2009) are one of the few who have addressed this point, suggesting that the low and high levels, while using distinct neural networks, work together, integrating their signals (p. 1633).

The second distinction, between internal and external focus, contrasts interior thoughts, feelings, experiences with external physical or visual events. This differs from the third distinction, between self and other, in that one can focus on one's own or others' internal states or one's own or others' external states. Fonagy and colleagues emphasize the importance of balancing an internal and external focus.

The third distinction, between self-oriented and other-oriented mentalization, is pivotal. As already noted, mentalizing can be about the self or about others. Taking Fonagy's view and sharpening it, I submit that mentalizing has to do with the ability to use what others think as part of one's own self-mentalizing. So, mentalizing about others and mentalizing about the self are not separate and distinct; they are integrally related to each other.

Using the mentalizing of others in your own self-mentalizing can be a matter of valuing someone else's mentalizing about general matters, or it can mean specifically valuing someone else's mentalizing about you. It does not necessarily mean that one accepts others' mentalizing as valid.

The fourth distinction, cognition and affect, distinguishes Fonagy's perspective from either the French psychosomatic or the cognitive science perspectives. It is consistent with recent views that reject the conventional distinction between cognition and affect and that highlight their interdependence through connectivity (Pessoa, 2008). As we will see, the concept of mentalized affectivity affirms the possibility of integrating cognition and affect. Indeed, the way I conceive the integration of cognition and affect ("affect-infused cognition") derives from psychoanalysis, and differs from the dominant model, where cognition presides over and subdues affect (discussed in Chapter 2).

Besides being comprehensive and integrative, mentalization theory is not simply an abstract point of view about the mind. It is the basis of an evidence-based approach to the treatment of borderline personality disorder (Bateman & Fonagy, 2006; Fonagy & Bateman, 2010). Mentalization-based therapy (MBT) is one of the few evidence-based psychoanalytic treatments, and deserves recognition for preserving psychoanalytic thinking in the current mental health world. In randomized controlled trials, Bateman and Fonagy (1999) have demonstrated that patients receiving MBT showed reduced depressive symptoms, fewer suicide attempts, fewer hospital stays, and better social functioning. Patients receiving MBT showed continued improvement 18 months posttreatment (Bateman & Fonagy, 2001). Moreover, in an 8-year follow-up study, patients receiving MBT still showed more improvement than a treatment-as-usual group (Bateman & Fonagy, 2008). MBT has been recognized internationally as a treatment for severe personality disorders.[8] It is currently being expanded to treat various other kinds of psychopathology, such as depression, trauma, addiction, and antisocial personality disorders, and is being used as a treatment for adults, children, adolescents, and families.

Fonagy has made an even larger claim about mentalization—that the "essence of psychotherapy is mentalizing" and that "psychotherapy enhances mentalization" (Fonagy, Bateman, & Luyten, 2012; also see Allen, Fonagy, & Bateman, 2008). Nevertheless, he urges caution about elevating mentalization to be the aim of therapy; rather, he claims that it mediates effectiveness by helping to build epistemic trust. In infants, we recall, epistemic trust renders one open and receptive to communication from caregivers, who thus initiate them into the world of culture. Without epistemic trust, psychotherapeutic interventions have little chance of being effective. In the context of psychotherapy, epistemic trust can be rekindled through the relationship to the therapist. As Fonagy concludes, "Put simply, the experience of feeling thought about in therapy

---

[8]MBT is currently in use in the following countries: Norway, Denmark, Sweden, Finland, Italy, Holland, Germany, Spain, Switzerland, Austria, the United Kingdom, the United States, Australia, New Zealand, Brazil, and Peru.

makes us feel safe enough to think about ourselves in relation to our world, and to learn something new about that world and how we operate in it" (Fonagy & Allison, 2014, p. 375). In this emerging account, the accent is on learning from experience, featuring the importance of learning about others and about the social realm.

MENTALIZING ABOUT MENTALIZATION

Thinking about mentalization inspires further mentalization, and I would like to pick up strands from the discussion so far, clarifying some points, considering where mentalization theory is heading, and specifying limitations that should be acknowledged. I have suggested that mentalization theory has moved in the direction of acknowledging the paradigm of communication. Communication is specific to humans and thus differs from attachment, which exists throughout the animal world. The communication paradigm is based on a constellation of ideas that I have already discussed (natural pedagogy, epistemic trust, and epistemic vigilance) and will discuss later (episodic memory, AM, and narrative).

According to the communication paradigm, our reliance on communication is a product of evolution, once humans began to live in larger groups bound by belief systems. Thus, some forms of psychopathology—like personality disorders—can be understood as breakdowns in communication. In Chapters 6 and 7, I discuss how communication can be improved through psychotherapy. Communication as a biological instinct should be distinguished from the hortatory everyday use of the term.

Using the communication paradigm as the basis of mentalization entails qualification of the meaning of attachment, but not a rejection of it. After all, psychotherapy is an experiment in activation of the attachment system, under controlled circumstances, so that mentalizing can emerge, be restored when lost, and be cultivated. The role of the therapist is to listen to and to mentalize about the patient. In one sense, the therapist's mentalizing serves to lead the patient to be able to see him- or herself more accurately. In another sense, the purpose of the therapist's mentalizing is to stimulate patients to mentalize for themselves, which would have to include the possibility of the therapist's mentalizing being corrected and altered by the patient. It can be helpful for therapists to mentalize about themselves. For example, a therapist might articulate his or her own thinking process in listening to and reacting to the patient. This can encourage a patient to think in a way that is less threatening than if the therapist directly describes what he or she thinks the patient is thinking. For patients who mentalize poorly, it can take a long time before they appreciate the value of doing so. For patients who are able to mentalize, therapy offers the experience of mentalizing together, spurring each party to take in and process how the other sees things. Finally, as I discuss in Chapters 6 and 7, there is the possibility of mutual mentalizing, where the therapist and patient mentalize in a collaborative way, where each makes a contribution to the whole process synergistically. (On this point, also see Tomasello, 2016, on the advantages of collaborative mentalizing for children's cultural learning.)

The role of the therapist is as both an attachment figure (which facilitates the expression of transference) and as a representative of social cognition. The attachment aspect reminds us that there is a personal, intimate quality to the relationship. Yet, it is mistaken to emphasize this aspect at the expense of the fact that the therapist–patient relationship is inescapably a social one, where the therapist hopes to improve the patient's general social cognition and the patient knows that he or she lacks knowledge about the therapist. Needless to say, some patients need more help with attachment-oriented relationships or with general social cognition, and they will bring varying capacities and preferences to the work. Distinguishing between these two realms, and not confusing them, is important and ought to become the subject of more attention in mentalization theory.

Another important and vexing question about mentalization concerns its relation to other familiar concepts such as empathy, psychological mindedness, and open-mindedness (Allen et al., 2008; Choi-Kain & Gunderson, 2008; Ensink & Mayes, 2010). The relation between empathy and mentalization is especially worth considering carefully. Allen and colleagues (2008) address this by proposing that empathy is a more narrow concept, although they acknowledge that ideas like "cognitive empathy" come closer to mentalization (Stueber's notion of "reenactive empathy" would be a related example). They take the position that empathy is only half the story—that it is concerned with others' mental states, not our own. Choi-Kain and Gunderson (2008) and Ensink and Mayes (2010) offer similar positions, which acknowledge the overlap between empathy and mentalization, but see empathy as more other-oriented.

But is it fair to claim that empathy must be strictly other-directed? The term "self-empathy" sounds awkward—the legacy of our cultural ambivalence toward paying attention to oneself, which, from Socrates on, affirms the value of seeking self-knowledge but remains wary of self-indulgence and narcissism. The philosopher Nancy Sherman has attempted to make the case for "self-empathy" as intelligible in the context of discussing veterans who are grappling with trauma, particularly "moral injury," where the suffering is self-caused rather than caused by another.[9] Sherman (2014) claims that self-empathy is the path of healing such suffering. It is not just a matter of being kind to or going easy on oneself; self-empathy requires something more, something like "fair self-assessment." Self-empathy encourages us to assume a perspective that is turned to the self but that sustains narrative distance. Sherman seems to be imagining a kind of objectivity, although she does not take up the crucial question of confirming that one's self-assessment is accurate. Sherman dwells on the benefits of self-empathy: that it helps us to be less burdened by adopting a less rigid standard of success and failure and that it weighs against self-destructive feelings. She regards self-empathy as fostering "self-reintegration" and the experience of "affectively alive ownership of past and future." In her account, self-empathy requires "self-friendship," a generosity of spirit that dovetails with the pursuit of self-knowledge.

Sherman (2014) extends her argument to psychotherapy in that self-empathy emerges from receiving empathy from a therapist. She also gives an example where a rape victim in a support group first experiences empathy in her reaction to other group members, which she then is able to apply to herself. Sherman's point of view fits well with my suggestion that mentalization promotes the ability to make use of others' point of view in order to better understand oneself. Sherman's point is that we can learn from others in the sense of doing for oneself what others have done for themselves. She does not specifically address my point that others' view of oneself can be taken up, reconciled against how one thinks of oneself, and then internalized.

So, empathy and mentalization are related concepts, especially insofar as mentalization relies on emotions. One can mentalize about other things—such as beliefs and values—but ultimately, mentalization in the context of psychotherapy has to involve emotions. Some readings of empathy seem to be closely tied to an intuitive responsiveness, or contagion, that has to exist uneasily with the emphasis Sherman places on self-empathy as perspective taking. Mentalization also requires such perspective taking. In mentalizing, beliefs are worn lightly, and we must be prepared to modify them as new evidence becomes available. Peirce's (1897) notion of "fallibilism" captures this aspect of mentalization: a humble, ongoing search to adjust and alter our beliefs. One assumes that in the future things will look different from how they do in the present, and one does not aspire to be self-reliant in a way that ignores the opportunity to learn from others.

It is mistaken to conjure the ideal mentalizer alone in a room by himself or herself; in its highest instantiation, mentalizing has to be

---

[9]For an elaboration of the idea of "moral injury," see Shay (2014).

welcoming toward mutual exchanges. The fact that the mentalizing of others is a spur to self-mentalize should not be taken to valorize individual mentalizing over collaborative mentalizing. Mentalization differs from psychoanalytic notions like insight or the observing ego precisely in having an intersubjective basis and in valuing social cognition.

Although it is crucial and wonderful to mentalize in life, we should not assume it comes naturally or easily to anyone. In other words, we ought to be careful to avoid the conceit that only borderline patients struggle to mentalize. We all struggle, and we all do so regularly. Indeed, we are often drawn to mentalize precisely where we realize we ought to have mentalized but failed to do so. This might happen, for example, if we do not linger with and struggle to make sense of aporetic emotions. So, I hesitate before the conclusion that the more we mentalize, the better, or that the need to mentalize is perpetual and constant. There is, perhaps, a low level of mentalization that is automatic, but the high level, our main concern in psychotherapy, is only relevant occasionally.

In truth, it is not desirable to mentalize all of the time. Therefore, it is a part of mentalizing to mentalize about whether to mentalize. Clearly, though, curtailing mentalizing is necessary at some moments, and knowing the limits of when to mentalize and when not to do so is a whole area that needs to be explored further. No justification exists for construing mentalization as more appropriate than spontaneity under some circumstances.

Mentalizing is often retrospective, rather than prospective. Thought can help us anticipate action, but it can also follow action. Mentalizing aids us in predicting what will happen, although there is research that questions our ability to use reflection in order to guide action directly (Mercier & Sperber, 2011). Significantly, mentalizing has a crucial role in making sense of the past, too. This will become clearer in the context of discussing mentalized affectivity and its connection to AM in the following section (and following chapter). The fact that there are limits to our ability to mentalize is important: it underscores its compatibility with the dynamic unconscious, as mental life is not conscious and threatening affects are banned from consciousness. In affirming our capacity to expand our conscious minds, mentalization theory does not presume that we are able to render the mind transparent.

The value of mentalization can be circumscribed: it is a means to an end, not an end in itself. Cultivating the capacity for mentalization, though, like contemplation itself, can be pleasurable and meaningful, and thus we should view it instrumentally or reduce its merit to practical benefit. We ought to embrace the challenge of striving to mentalize emotions as a path that brings rewards and equips us to resist perils and to experience life as governed in some measure by agency.

WHAT IS MENTALIZED AFFECTIVITY?

How can mentalization be enhanced by psychotherapy? The answer can be found in the concept of mentalized affectivity, which "generates the insight into emotional experience that psychotherapy provides" (Fonagy et al., 2012).

Mentalized affectivity is the part of mentalization theory that encompasses the diverse aspects of experiencing emotions that we have reviewed in Part I—identifying, modulating, and expressing emotions—not just in the present tense, but through recall as well. All forms of psychotherapy regard emotions as part of the healing process, and many forms have begun to center on the notion of emotion regulation. Almost all psychopathology has an aspect of emotional suffering, and so the aim of therapy is often to help patients experience and work with their emotions more effectively. Given the background of mentalization theory in psychoanalysis, there are some specific points that distinguish it from other kinds of psychotherapy. The stance psychoanalysis takes on emotions is different from the basic emotions paradigm, which sees emotions as immediate, short-lived, and transparent. Understanding emotions is tricky, and the process unavoidably involves self-deception and misunderstanding. Emotions themselves exist in disguised and combined forms; therefore, it takes work to make sense of them.

Mentalized affectivity overlaps with emotion regulation insofar as it involves modulating and crafting emotions to be more precise. However, it is not just another fancy term for the same process. Mentalized affectivity is based on the recognition that emotion regulation is affected by personality style, values, and most importantly, AM. A stimulus–response paradigm, which is typically assumed in research on emotion regulation, does not acknowledge the extent to which our present experience is mediated by the past. So, a helpful way to think of mentalized affectivity is as joining the domains of emotion regulation and AM.

Mentalized affectivity aims not to modulate and transform our emotions, but to reevaluate them by means of reexperiencing them with some perspective. Incorporating AM is necessary in order to be able to fathom and articulate complex emotional experience. Indeed, we have already seen that the self is implicated in identifying, modulating, and expressing emotions. We turn to the past not to seek "buried treasure," but as a way to understand how it continues to influence the present and point to the future. Memories of the past can be individual or cultural. It is widely appreciated that individual memories are constantly being updated and reconstituted; as Winter (2012) highlights, cultural memories and narratives are equally changeable.

It is, perhaps, less obvious, and more challenging, to consider how turning to the past actually alters and counterbalances our memories of the past. For example, a patient who came to treatment furious at his mother for denying abusive behavior on the part of the patient's sibling for a long time recalled only negative memories of his relationship with her. Toward the end of the treatment, he produced entirely new memories in which it was evident that his mother had been under great stress. His mentalizing of his relationship with her altered what had been predominantly painful memories; it also made it possible for him to regulate his current interactions with his mother, where he felt relief from making the choice to establish firmer boundaries between them and greater psychic distance.

Mentalized affectivity can impart new insights, but it can also become deployed as an ongoing capacity, providing hope that whatever happens in life, one will have ways to make sense of and deal with it. Ideally, mentalized affectivity fuels the experience that our life belongs to us and that generosity to self and others will prevail.

MEASURING REFLECTIVE FUNCTION AND MENTALIZED AFFECTIVITY

Our field has developed and tested ways of assessing reflective function, the operationalized version of mentalization, and, more recently, mentalized affectivity. The first measure of reflective function was the Reflective Functioning Scale (RFS; Fonagy, 1996), which uses a scoring procedure based on transcripts of the Adult Attachment Interviews (AAI; George, Kaplan, & Main, 1985). The RFS is coded with an 11-point scale, ranging from antireflective (–1) to exceptionally reflective (9). It has produced intriguing findings, such as that mentalization is the missing link that transmits attachment security from parents to their children, and that there is a deficit of mentalization in borderline personality disorder, but this can be altered by psychotherapy (see Taubner et al., 2013, for a comprehensive review of the RFS). However, the evaluation of the transcripts and the considerable training needed for coders makes this a time-consuming measure. Thus, Fonagy and colleagues (2016) created the Reflective Function Questionnaire (the RFQ-54, with 54 questions, and a shorter version, the RFQ-8, with 8 questions). The measure has an internal consistency of alpha = .70.

The RFQ relies on self-report, which, as Fonagy and colleagues (2016) well recognize, is challenging, since it means that poor mentalizers are asked to attempt to mentalize (objectively) about themselves.[10] The RFQ-54 poses questions that combine feeling and thinking; a few questions focus on specific emotions (like anger), others on curiosity about emotions and the struggle to make sense of emotions. The RFQ-8 has two questions about general feelings, two on anger, one on insecurity, one on thought, and two on action. Both versions of this measure include emotions but have a broader focus.

The RFQ can be used to help discern vulnerability to psychopathology. As Fonagy and colleagues (2016) propose, the RFQ reveals two different kinds of impairment in mentalizing: hypomentalizing and hypermentalizing. Hypomentalizing is characterized by concreteness and the prementalizing style of "psychic equivalence," where one assumes that if something is in one's mind, it must be in the mind of others. This kind of mentalizing has been linked to borderline personality disorder, eating disorders, and depression. Hypermentalizing denotes a pseudo style of mentalizing in which expression outweighs content—that is, it is excessive in nature. The deficient quality of this mentalizing can be obscured by a false confidence gained from its quantity. Interestingly, Sharp and Venta (2012) have found that in adolescents, hypermentalizing is strongly associated with borderline traits. Both hypomentalizing and hypermentalizing can be contrasted to genuine mentalizing, where there is a respect for the opacity of minds but a curiosity about fathoming the inner worlds of oneself or others. Fonagy and colleagues refer to the sense of autonomy, agency, and freedom to explore mental states that underlie genuine mentalizing.

Two factors are introduced in the RFQ measure to give greater specificity to the reflective function construct: a scale based on certainty (RFQ_C) and uncertainty (RFQ_U) of mental states. For example, certainty would be indicated through disagreement with statements like "I don't always know why I do what I do," and uncertainty in agreement with statements like "Sometimes I do things without really knowing why." Not agreeing (or low agreement) with certainty suggests hypermentalizing, whereas readily agreeing (or high agreement) would be consistent with genuine mentalizing, the ability to discern opacity in mental states. Extremes in uncertainty were intended to assess hypomentalizing, whereas some recognition of uncertainty would be consistent with genuine mentalizing, the ability to discern opacity in mental

---

[10]Fonagy and Luyten are in the process of developing a Q-sort measure of reflective function that would avoid depending on self-report in favor of therapists' ratings of patients.

states. The results of three studies are reported. In the first, the RFQ_U scale is superior to the RFQ_C scale in capturing problems that occur in borderline personality disorder; in the second study, the RFQ_U was significantly associated with clinical status; and in the third study, where parental reflective function was expected to mediate the relationship between reflective function and infant attachment security, the RFQ_C, but not the RFQ_U, correlated with security. Although these findings are not fully consistent, they are fascinating in terms of explicating the notion of aporetic emotions. In some ways, it seems, it is desirable to acknowledge that one is confused about what one feels; however, it can be a warning sign not to be able to move beyond this state.

An alternative way to measure reflective function has been introduced by Fertuck, Mergenthaler, Target, Levy, and Clarkin (2012). Rather than a narrative-based assessment, this scale (the Computerized Reflective Functioning Scale [CRF]) uses computerized text analysis, which identifies linguistic markers of reflective function. It relies on finding meaning in the quantity and frequency of word usage and making inferences about individuals and groups based on the language they use through a content analysis: 54 linguistic markers of high-reflective-function language were identified, and the study demonstrated that associations between the CRF and reflective function were significant in both a clinical sample (patients diagnosed with borderline personality disorder) and a nonclinical sample of adults. The authors see the computerized approach as offering a less cumbersome way to assess reflective function that potentially allows us to glimpse mechanisms of symptom and personality change. Although this scale needs further validation, it is specifically devised to be used on clinical samples, unlike the RFS.

Given my interest specifically in mentalizing emotions, my research group has developed a scale that tries to operationalize and measure mentalized affectivity. We hope that the scale will enable us to carry out an assessment of (and serve as a continuing means to assess) the ability to engage with and perhaps improve mentalized affectivity. Our aim in developing the Mentalized Affectivity Scale (MAS) was to broaden the territory of emotion regulation scales, including but differentiating the spheres of identifying, modulating, and expressing emotions, and welcoming emotions that are remembered. We also wished to explore the notion of aporetic emotions. Most importantly, we were interested in investigating whether and to what degree our emotional reactions are governed by history and experience. The MAS is a 60-item self-report measure. So far, the measure has been administered to over 2,000 subjects via a website where participants took a variety of psychological tests on music, personality, and social psychology.

Psychometric analyses showed that the measure successfully delineates the three components, identifying, modulating (here termed "processing"), and expressing emotions, as independent of each other. Our intention was to link this to basic tendencies (such as personality traits), situational factors (such as traumatic events), and well-being. Results showed that mentalized affectivity, and specifically a high level of processing/modulating, predicted life satisfaction beyond demographics, personality, and situational factors. One interesting finding is that scoring high on identifying and low on processing seems to link to self-reports of psychopathology. Preliminary findings from retrospective accounts suggest that identifying and expressing emotions are elevated for those participants who are in therapy compared to those who are not. Further research will test this finding using longitudinal designs, especially the role of processing emotions in therapy. For readers who would like to learn about the MAS in more detail, see the Appendix and also a research article from my lab (Greenberg et al., 2017).

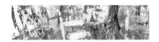 CHAPTER 5

Cultivating Mentalized Affectivity

Emotional experience is the first step towards a thought. At
the end of the road, we find thinking . . . in psychoanalysis
we have to keep the emotional experience in the mind and
to reflect on it, to transform it without evacuating it, to
be aware of it, without either being overwhelmed by it or
murdering it. So thought cannot be dissociated from pain,
suffering, pleasure, ecstasy.
—ANDRÉ GREEN, "The Primordial Mind
and the Work of the Negative" (1998)

Although mentalized affectivity grows out of the mentalization literature, it overlaps with emergent concepts in the study of emotions.
Like emotional intelligence, mentalized affectivity has to do with using
emotions well and with acknowledging how using emotions links with
a good life. Emotional intelligence emerged as an effort to distinguish
and articulate a kind of intelligence different from cognitive intelligence.
According to Goleman (1995) emotional intelligence has to do with "self-
control, zeal and persistence, and the ability to motivate oneself" (p. xii).
Thus, the concept syncs naturally with culturally normative preferences:
it resonates with the Protestant work ethic, particularly with its evolving American construals, and has been widely embraced in classrooms
and in the business world. Moreover, it is apparent that emotional intelligence is closely tied to the capacity for emotion regulation, as more
scientific descriptions of emotional intelligence have pointed out (Mayer
& Salovey, 1997). Several measures of emotional intelligence have been
developed (Schutte et al., 1998).

As I have argued in Chapter 2, the concept of emotion regulation has a normative bias that ought to make us cautious about ascribing universality to it. Emotional intelligence and emotion regulation are valuable concepts, but they downplay differences in beliefs, values, and history and, ultimately, can be too easily applied (even unintentionally) as a way to reward privilege. As Illouz (2007, 2008) argues, emotional intelligence harnesses emotions to problem solving; it produces the formalization and codification of competence that promotes social benefit and social capital within the system of contemporary capitalism.

Mentalized affectivity aims to incorporate the capacity to identify, modulate, and express emotions, and to negotiate how emotions are inevitably social and yet permit an opportunity for freedom, creative self-expression, and resistance to social norms. Mentalized affectivity promotes the challenge of reflecting on emotions, recognizing but not necessarily deferring to established cultural beliefs.

What makes mentalized affectivity a unique concept is that, by definition, it construes the past, both individual and cultural, as mediating present and future experience. Although some versions of emotional intelligence and emotion regulation offer complex descriptions of the sequence of appraising and expressing emotions, they mainly focus on the present experience of the individual. In contrast, mentalized affectivity depends on utilizing AM.

In Chapter 4, I pointed out that the concept of mentalized affectivity brings together aspects of the separate domains of emotion regulation and AM. More attention needs to be paid to the relation between AM and emotion regulation, as Pasupathi (2003) has observed. There are indications that this is starting to occur—for example, a recent study by Selcuk, Zayas, Günaydin, Hazan, and Kross (2012) looks at how the mental representation of attachment figures in memory facilitates the regulation of emotions elicited by internally generated stressors and makes a plea for further study. Let us take a closer look at the literature on AM, narrative, and self.

AUTOBIOGRAPHICAL MEMORY/NARRATIVE/SELF

The subfield of AM (AM) is growing, as documented in Figure 5.1. Although autobiographical memory (AM) itself represents an entire area of study, our focus will emphasize how it is related to mentalized affectivity.

We carry our history with us in the form of our AM, which in turn contributes to our experience of emotions and our sense of being a coherent and continuous entity (Conway, 2005). Many researchers

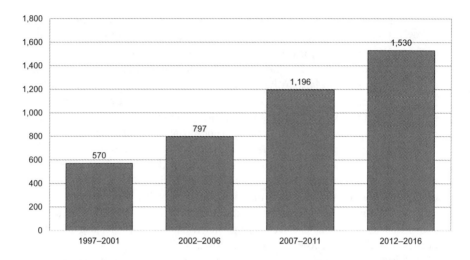

FIGURE 5.1. Proliferating references to "autobiographical memory" in Psyc-INFO (1997–2016).

are intrigued that AM influences and is influenced by the self; however, other researchers are more skeptical about linking memory to the self—for example, Rubin (2012), who argues that it is premature to understand AM with reference to the self, given that we do not know so much about the self. It is helpful, perhaps, to begin by placing AM in a larger context.

AM begins in childhood. Some researchers have focused on different moments of development, like childhood amnesia or "the reminiscence bump." Fivush (2012) offers a compelling developmental point of view that highlights the unfolding of a personal timeline in childhood (roughly, from the end of preschool years), which establishes what she terms "a subjective perspective." A subjective perspective has three elements: (1) the representation of the self; (2) the understanding that the self has internal states (thoughts, emotions, beliefs, desires) that are coherently linked to behavior; and (3) the understanding that others also have internal states and that others' internal states may be the same as or different from one's own (Fivush, 2012, p. 232). Fivush is not primarily concerned with emotions, but her view fits well with mentalization theory and with mentalized affectivity, as she stresses that the subjective perspective helps us tune into and predict our own and others' behavior.

How is AM related to the self? One important proposal is found in Conway and Pleydell-Pearce (2000) and Conway (2005), who describe a "self-memory system," which comprises AM, as well as the "working self," which is made up of goals and self-images. The "working self" also maintains the coherence of a person's goals, in part by regulating how events are remembered. AM contains a record of the goal system and serves as a basis for the development of new goals (Conway, 2009). According to this proposal, we use the past to guide us but also to mark how we might want to change. As Berntsen and Rubin (2012) observe, AM helps to reduce self-discrepancy, where one faces up to disparities between the actual and possible self.

Bluck, Alea, Habermas, and Rubin (2005) delineate three functions of AM: directive (using the past to guide the present as well as the future), self (helping us sustain a sense of self-continuity over time), and social (helping us to develop and nurture social relationships and intimacy). Thus, AM is invoked not just to recall the past, but to aid us in dealing with the present and anticipating the future. AM enables us to time travel mentally, and thus leads to the expansion of consciousness. It serves multiple purposes for the self, but not necessarily restricted to the self, such as contributing to the flourishing of social life.

Habermas (2015) stresses the point that AM helps to foster narratives. Narratives have two functions: communication of events and their evaluation. Habermas specifically argues that narratives are successful or not depending on their use of emotion. Correspondingly, he suggests that problems with narrating AM result in various forms of psychopathology, including personality disorders. Habermas appreciates the interpersonal and social potential of AM, as it enables self-understanding but also mutual understanding between self and others (also see Conway & Jobson, 2012; Moscovitch, 2012; Pillemer & Kuwabara, 2015). In recognizing how AM infuses personal, historical, and cultural dimensions, Habermas's view, which features the contribution of AM to communication, fits wells with the idea of mentalized affectivity. While autobiographical memories are often woven into narratives, it remains unclear how to judge such narratives, such as in situations in which the self and others are in conflict. For example, it is not difficult to imagine that one might feel one's narrative is coherent and accurate, while someone else might be threatened by it; or that one (defensively) regards one's own narrative as coherent and accurate, while another wishes to question it. In addition, there are unresolved issues about the degree to which narratives have holes that cannot and should not be filled, and whether a lack of seamlessness actually contributes to authenticity. I would argue, in fact, that in the autobiographical memoirs we have encountered, authenticity is established, in part, by *not* obscuring gaps in the narrative.

Damasio (1994, 1999, 2010) offers a neuroscientific view of AM that leads to the autobiographical self. Damasio (1999) has argued that the elaboration of AM is a key to "extended consciousness," which "occurs when working memory holds in place, simultaneously, *both* a particular object *and* the autobiographical self" (p. 222). More specifically, he has argued that the ventromedial prefrontal cortex plays a critical role in terms of triggering somatic responses from what he terms "secondary inducers." Secondary inducers are "entities generated by the recall of a personal or hypothetical emotional event, or perceiving a primary inducer that generates 'thoughts' and 'memories' about the inducer." Primary inducers are stimuli that unconditionally or through learning produce negative or positive somatic states—like fearing a snake (or a stimulus that is predictive of a snake or even relevant semantic knowledge). Patients with impaired ventromedial prefrontal cortex can experience an emotion like fear through primary inducers, but not through secondary inducers—a handicap that interferes with normal decision making. The as-if loop of "somatic markers," Damasio argues, is important because it allows us to rehearse and to be able to make more precise emotional responses.

Damasio's work provides intriguing evidence for the importance of emotions and their profound relation to the self. In his most recent book (Damasio, 2010), he argues that the self has evolved in order to aid "life regulation," and that it emerges from the brain stem, not just the neocortex. The self can be defined both in terms of being a knower (and protagonist) of experience and as an object. Damasio delineates three kinds of self, which are connected to emotions: (1) the proto-self, which is born from primordial (spontaneous) feelings and is manifested through the mapping of the body; (2) the core self, which allows the protagonist to feel (basic emotions) and to respond and attend to objects in the present; and (3) the autobiographical self, which transcends homeostasis to include "social homeostasis," that is, socially mediated emotions that aim at well-being and that encompass past, present, and future. The autobiographical self serves to link current experience to patterns that can be recalled in memory. Of course, lots of unanswered questions might be posed: does everyone have an autobiographical self in Damasio's sense, or is it an achievement that few people attain? Can therapy help to forge an autobiographical self (and is this an aim of all therapy)?

AM, the ability to recollect personally experienced past events, is essential to human functioning; it contributes to one's sense of self, and to the ability to remain focused on goals in light of past decisions and history. Some forms of emotional regulation, therefore, can be understood as aiming to add more specificity to one's AM. Research has shown that individuals suffering from depression (and also trauma) tend to have overly general autobiographic memories (for a review of these studies, see Williams et al., 2007). Moreover, as Brown, Kouri, and Superka (2015) observe, improvement in autobiographical specificity is useful as a marker of therapeutic recovery. It would be mistaken, however, to assume that autobiographical memories are necessarily beneficial: Philippe, Koestner, Lecours, Beaulieu-Pelletier, and Bois (2011) demonstrate how autobiographical memories concerning the thwarting of one's needs has an impact on current experiences of emotions, calling for future study of this point.

The ability to recall specific memories is clearly not just relevant for clinical populations. The arousal level elicited by general memories is higher than that elicited when recalling a more specific memory (Philippot, Baeyens, & Douilliez, 2006). Thus, the ability to recall a specific past memory in order to place a current emotion in an autobiographic context may help to reduce arousal level, making it more tolerable, reducing the pressure to act on it, and modulating it through the use of strategies such as those detailed in the process model described in Chapter 2. Wheeler, Stuss, and Tulving (1997) have termed this ability "autonoetic (*self-knowing*) consciousness."

Wheeler and his colleagues (1997) remind us of a relevant quotation from William James describing the act of recalling a past experience: "remembrance is like a direct feeling; its object is suffused with a warmth and an intimacy to which no object of mere conception ever attains" (p. 239). These authors argue that the ability to travel back in time is an expression of episodic memory and is related to, but not the same as, autobiographic memory. The quotation from James helps to clarify this distinction in the sense that this type of memory is not merely cognitive. It entails a reexperiencing of the past event and is infused with affect, albeit usually less intensely than the original experience. This capacity, Wheeler and colleagues argue, is central to our humanity. They maintain, in addition, that it is important to keep in mind a coherent representation of our past and who we are, but to be able to move forward into the future: "Indeed, it is difficult to imagine that an individual could mentally prepare oneself for any kind of future undertaking without some representation of self as a stable entity that endures over time" (p. 335).

The context in which this mental time travel occurs is important. Sutin and Gillath (2009) demonstrate in an attachment priming study that participants in the "secure" condition self-reported more coherent memories than those in the "insecure" condition. Moreover, priming attachment insecurity actually had the effect of decreasing memory coherence. Thus, for mentalized affectivity to enhance one's sense of self and elicit more coherent episodic memories, it is optimal for it to occur within a safe and caring interpersonal context. Under such conditions, we can hypothesize, emotional memories can also be subject to modification, refinement, and revised meaning.

The process of reflecting on emotions provides some distance from the intensified affect. In a recent imaging study that attempted to examine the neural underpinnings of emotion regulation, distinguishing between mindful introspection and more cognitive reflection, Herwig, Kaffenberger, Jäncke, and Brühl (2010) divided 30 subjects into three conditions: cognitive self-reflection ("think"), emotion-introspection ("feel"), and indifference ("neutral"). The results showed distinct but overlapping activation of the cortex; however, the left amygdala was activated in think condition but deactivated in feel condition—suggesting an attenuated influence of arousal. As these authors suggest, "making oneself aware of how one feels may lead to an inner distancing from these feelings and thus may represent an important strategy for the self-regulation of emotions" (p. 738).

AM and the self are connected: the self is constituted through memories, and memories are understood from the vantage point of the self. I have addressed views that defend the potential for autobiographical memories to become an autobiographical self through narrative. Some researchers have placed the emphasis more on "self-defining memories," rather than narrative per se. Moreover, it seems worthwhile to acknowledge that not all autobiographical memories are voluntary; some autobiographical memories are unbidden or may be out of our awareness.

Keep in mind that research linking AM and the self is not well established. It seems plausible to imagine that AM and the autobiographical self overlap, but the case for this claim depends on formulating testable hypotheses and predictions. Concerned about the gap between theory and research, Prebble, Addis, and Tippett (2013), distinguish between subjective and objective, and between the present and temporally extended aspects of the self. They argue that self-awareness in the present moment is a vital precursor to autonoetic consciousness (the recollective experience of perceiving the self as extended in time) and episodic memory. Prebble and colleagues build this argument by taking account of two competing theories of AM. The first, by Tulving and colleagues, emphasizes the link between episodic memory and the subjective aspects of the self. Episodic memory can be contrasted with semantic memory in that the former relies on autonoetic consciousness, while the latter does not. Semantic memory relies instead on noetic consciousness, that is, objectively thinking about something one knows. In contrast, episodic memory presumes a self, as Tulving (2005) suggests in claiming there can be no time travel without a traveler.

The second theory, by Conway and colleagues, maintains that abstracted, semanticized forms of AM are necessary in order to construct a stable mental representation of the self. Episodic memory, in their account, provides accurate record keeping, but it dissipates quickly.

Thus, episodic memory can be regarded as the base of AM, but it is in need of the conceptual organization that the self-memory system provides. What is distinctive about Conway and colleagues' view is that there is a bidirectional relation between memory and the self: autobiographical memories help to construct the self, and the resulting conceptual self influences how the memories are used (Conway, 2005). Prebble and colleagues (2013) attempt to reconcile the difference between Tulving and Conway by affirming that the subjective experience of the self is a precondition for episodic AM (and the sense of phenomenological continuity) but also valuing the conceptual, semanticized parts of AM, which aid in the formation and sustaining of a coherent self-concept both in the present and over time. They conclude that there is reason to support the link between AM and the self, although more research needs to be done.[1]

Mahr and Csibra (2017) consider episodic memory from the perspective of communication. They propose that rather than aiming to predict the future, episodic memory grounds veridical beliefs, helping us to take responsibility for beliefs by seeking to support them. They contrast this "epistemic generosity" with the more circumscribed function of semantic memory. Ultimately, epistemic memory serves to enhance individuals by strengthening their capacity for epistemic vigilance as well as spreading cooperation among humans. While not emphasized in Mahr and Csibra, the positive attributes of episodic memory are germane to the therapeutic process.

In short, mentalized affectivity relies on AM as an aid to help us to define ourselves on an ongoing basis. It requires that we embrace a deeper exploration of the meaning of emotional experience in the context of our life, history, and environment. Mentalized affectivity entails an openness to knowing, amending, correcting, and rendering emotional experience into a more articulated form. This articulation can certainly prompt engagement in the writing, editing, and rewriting of one's autobiography and ideas about the self. Even as we complete the "latest edition," we are already in the process of preparing and writing the next version. A wonderful example of this is seen in the work of Oliver Sacks, who wrote two memoirs, kept over 1,000 diaries, completed multiple books, and continued writing moving self-reflections on his life until his death.

---

[1]It is important to acknowledge that evolutionary psychologists have expressed skepticism about the self; for example, Kurzban and Aktipis (2007) reject the concept in favor of the "social cognitive interface," which they liken to being a "press secretary." They make no room for the agentive self, the key concept in my thinking. Klein (2012) offers a different perspective, not wanting to abandon the ontological self, although it cannot be studied scientifically.

SACKS RESTRAINED

Oliver Sacks was a neurologist by training and was a devoted and extraordinarily sensitive clinician: "I have never seen a patient who didn't teach
me something new, or stir in me new feelings and new trains of thought"
(2015e, p. 227). He was not a researcher, and forthrightly documents
his failed efforts in that domain, but he maintained broad interests and
kept current with neuroscientific developments. Sacks's case studies
often included a personal element, which helped him win new audiences
for popular science writing. In addition, he wrote two autobiographies,
Uncle Tungsten (2001) and *On the Move* (2015e).

The two memoirs were written 14 years apart, although the former
was long in gestation, and they cover consecutive parts of Sacks's life—
Uncle Tungsten (*UT*) from early childhood to adolescence, *On the Move*
(*OM*) from early adulthood to old age. Many of Sacks's interests and
preoccupations remain the same: "metals, plants, and numbers" (*UT*,
p. 32). Yet, there is something extraordinarily different about the two
books. In *UT*, Sacks presents himself as a science nerd who was dramatically affected by being sent away from London during World War
II because of the bombing; in *OM*, we encounter an adventurous soul—
emigrating to North America, riding his motorcycle solo throughout the
American West, smashing weightlifting records, indulging in drugs, and
beginning to follow his own star as a physician and writer. Most importantly, Sacks reveals that he was gay and openly discusses his lifelong
struggle to connect with others, culminating at the end of his life in finding a fulfilling love relationship.

The first memoir, *UT*, is restrained, documenting young Oliver as
a studious experimenter in love with chemistry, especially the history of
chemistry, which he duplicates in a small room in his parents' home in
London. At the end of the memoir, it is unclear where Sacks is heading.
The second memoir, *OM*, is overflowing, documenting Sacks's rebel-
liousness, which led him to the United States, and his convoluted path
to becoming a writer on a wide range of neurological phenomena and
disorders. Movingly, the second memoir ends with falling in love and
partnering for the first time in his life. Although Sacks was in psychoanalysis at the time he wrote *UT*, this does not come up at any point in
the narrative. His relationship with his analyst is a subtle but crucial
theme in *OM*.

Sacks was in psychoanalysis with the same analyst, Leonard Shengold, for almost 50 years. Yes, 50 years! Was his analysis a factor that
might account for the difference between the two works, and for the
loosening up, the coming into himself, and his remarkable flourishing?
Perhaps, but Sacks's disclosure of his sexual orientation is also a measure of changes that occurred in the culture. Indeed, Sacks makes sure

to remind us that "it was not easy, or safe, to be an open or practicing homosexual in the London of the 1950s" (*OM,* p. 38). To what extent Sacks's evolution had to do with his analysis is a matter for speculation. I would argue, though, that there is an increase in mentalized affectivity between the two works. Even if we cannot know whether his analysis was responsible for this change, it is hard to believe that it did not contribute in a facilitative and salutary way.

I focus on these memoirs to provide detail and insight concerning mentalized affectivity as it manifests itself embedded in an actual life. The Sacks whom we encounter is adept at identifying emotions, struggles with modulating them, and is inhibited in expressing them. His autobiographical memories serve to forge a creative autobiographical narrative and autobiographical self.

Sacks begins *UT* with the association between his childhood memories and metals. It turns out, he means this both literally (given his love of chemistry) and symbolically (given that he associates metals with various family members). He recalls his mother's gold wedding ring and her showing him how heavy gold was in comparison to other metals. His mother also noted how soft gold was, and thus how it could be combined with other metals. Sacks also links his mother to diamonds, an extremely hard material that was cold to the touch, as his mother explained to him. Heavy, soft, but hard and cold—the metaphors do not add up neatly.

Sacks's relationship to his family was enormously affected by a trauma that befell him at 6 years old, when, because of the bombing of London during World War II, he was sent off to a boarding school outside the city. There he recalls being bullied and beaten severely, for instance, when he accidentally wet his bed (p. 29). His parents, both doctors, remained in London in order to work. Sacks explains how his relationship to his mother was changed by this experience: he became unable to respond to her and rejected Judaism, a contrast to his pleasant earlier memories of being held and kissed by his mother as he fell asleep on the Sabbath (p. 25). On the one hand, we can surmise that the normal separation-individuation process was interrupted when Sacks was sent away (however much it was a reasonable protective decision on the part of his parents). On the other hand, Sacks clearly felt that both of his parents were preoccupied with their own work over and above the exigencies of wartime. Tellingly, Sacks remembers being curious and asking his parents questions, only to be given answers that were completely over his head (p. 10).

Sacks was often brought along with his father, a general practitioner, on calls to patients. His mother, who had been trained as a surgeon but become an obstetrician, encouraged him to dissect malformed fetuses, which she had brought home for this purpose, when he was at the tender age of 11 years old. Sacks found the latter experience distressing, although he did not express this; nor did his mother seem to take note of it.

At one point, Sacks casually but decisively comments that his parents seemed to be more interested in their patients than in their children (p. 238). Yet, Sacks affectionately portrays the complexity of his mother's character, noting that she was shy and not very social but capable of being exuberant and flamboyant, and sees his own character as similar (p. 237). Sacks enumerates the specific qualities he admired most about his mother—her ability to concentrate, her love of structure, and her love of her garden—all of which he sees himself as having internalized.

Sacks identifies his father in terms of metal too: his mother, his three older brothers, and he had brass menorahs for Hanukkah, while his father's was silver. Almost as a passing thought, Sacks informs us that his father was "not given to emotion or intimacy" (p. 91). Yet, they experienced closeness when swimming together, which became a lifelong passion for Sacks. Sacks was strongly influenced by his father in his work, noting that his father's view of the practice of medicine was that it was not about diagnosis and "had to be seen and understood in the context of patients' lives, the particularities of their personalities, their feelings, their reactions" (p. 93). That Sacks was headed to a career in medicine was a foregone conclusion, as his two older brothers took this same path. That Sacks chose to become a neurologist is significant, as that actually had been his father's first career plan. At one point, Sacks hesitates about becoming a doctor and contemplates the appeal of botany because plants "do not have feelings" (p. 241).

Sacks muses about his two older brothers' decision to become doctors and notes with "sadness" that his brother David's true love was music, and Marcus's was languages (p. 186). Sacks's other brother, Michael, was troubled and became psychotic after being bullied at school, and was eventually diagnosed as schizophrenic. Sacks unsparingly admits how disturbing it was to witness what happened to his brother, propelling him to withdraw into science and away from the brother whom he feared. On a deeper level, Sacks reveals his own fear of becoming schizophrenic, a not uncommon experience for siblings. Sacks's position as the youngest of four boys was an advantage in fostering his scientific interests, but perhaps also a factor in his sense that his parents had many other priorities.

The wealth of meaningful relationships with extended family members—especially aunts and uncles—is a striking part of Sacks's family life. Indeed, the memoir's title refers to Sacks's uncle Dave, his mother's brother, who combined his love of science with a commercial business that produced lightbulbs. Sacks spent hours there, exposed to various kinds of metals and technologies, free to learn and experiment. The larger, symbolic meaning of tungsten is apparent in the association that Sacks provides: being "stable in a precarious world" (p. 39). The stability that Sacks experienced through his extended family seems, at least to some degree, to have compensated for what he did not receive from his parents.

A good deal of the narrative in *UT* is taken up by Sacks's love of chemistry. He voices his admiration for the merger of literary and scientific thinking in the 19th century, contrasting this to the current divide between the "two cultures" described by Snow (1959). Although *UT* dwells on Sacks's specialized scientific interests, there are glimpses into Sacks's own personality. For example, in the context of reviewing the poet-chemist Humphrey Davy's many discoveries, Sacks concludes that "it was Davy's personality that appealed to me—not modest, like Schelle, not systematic, like Lavoisier, but filled with exuberance and enthusiasm of a boy, with a wonderful adventurousness and sometimes dangerous impulsiveness—he was always at the point of going too far—and it was this which captured my imagination above all" (p. 131). Needless to say, Sacks identifies with Davy, and gently introduces us to a side of himself that is not well represented in *UT,* but is at the heart of *OM.*

Indeed, one of Sacks's favorite quotations about himself from a teacher, cited in both *UT* and *OM*, was "Sacks will go far if he does not go too far" (*UT*, p. 140; *OM,* p. 7). Sacks's impulsiveness is more in evidence in *OM* than in *UT.* Perhaps we can discern a tendency to go too far in Sacks's obsessive interests, but there is some irony here. The rejoinder that comes to mind to the teacher's remark is that Sacks went so far because he was willing to go too far.

In his early life, Sacks presents himself as a loner, as socially awkward and anxious. He chronicles his hypochondria and traces a sense of "fear and superstition" to his nightmare experience at the boarding school, which left as a residue the feeling that "some special awfulness might be reserved for me, and that this might descend at any moment" (p. 235). Sacks documents his various phobias: afraid that horses "might bite me with their large teeth; afraid of crossing the road, especially after our dog, Greta, was killed by a motorbike; afraid of other children, who (if nothing else) would laugh at me; afraid of stepping on the cracks between paving stones; and afraid, above all, of disease, of death" (p. 236). His investment in the natural world seems inversely related to his withdrawal from the social world.[2] Eventually, Sacks's commitment

---

[2] Sacks had a neurological condition, prosopagnosia (or face blindness), which causes impairment in the recognition of faces, and which might have contributed to his difficulty with social engagement.

to becoming a chemist wanes, as he hungers for "the human, the personal," that which had eluded him, and he finds himself newly attracted to "personal narratives and journals" (pp. 276–277). *UT* concludes uncertainly with Sacks entering adolescence. The final paragraph of the memoir culminates dramatically with a series of seven sentences that end with question marks.

SACKS REDUX: UNRESTRAINED

OM begins with a brief acknowledgment of Sacks's traumatic boarding school experience but quickly moves on from there. This new phase of his life is accompanied by a new style of self-presentation. His love of motorcycles figures as importantly in this volume as his love of chemistry did in *UT*. A major new trauma then befalls Sacks when his father betrays his confidence and tells his mother that he is gay. Her reaction: "You are an abomination. . . . I wish you had never been born" (pp. 9–10). Surprisingly, Sacks leans in the direction of being apologetic for this vile reaction: "My mother did not mean to be cruel, to wish me dead. She was suddenly overwhelmed, I now realize, and she probably regretted her words or perhaps partitioned them off in a closeted part of her mind" (p. 11). (Using "closeted" here seems strangely appropriate.) Yet, Sacks well understands the monumental impact it had for his mother to reject him for his sexual orientation: "But her words haunted me for much of my life and played a major part in inhibiting and injecting with guilt what should have been a free and joyous expression of sexuality" (p. 11). Sacks is not exaggerating on this point, as he later divulges that he went for 35 years without having sex after a brief fling at the age of 40 (p. 203). It is endearing to encounter the integrity and strength it takes to muster as much vulnerability as Sacks does in *OM*.

It is hugely to Sacks's credit that he can honestly acknowledge the profound and deleterious effect his mother's reaction had on him and, at the same time, emphasize how important a person she was in his life. Indeed, their bond is portrayed more positively in *OM* than in *UT* (possibly influenced by her death). He sees himself as her favorite son (p. 61). Moreover, he describes his mother's death as "the most devastating loss of my life—the loss of the deepest and perhaps, in some sense, the realest relation of my life" (p. 193). In *OM*, Sacks is also generous to his father, proudly recalling that he still made house calls when he was in his 90s, and belatedly coming to the realization in reviewing old letters that his parents cared about him deeply in their own way.

Overall, *OM* depicts a rocky road with the backdrop of the boarding school trauma, Sacks's struggle to feel good about being gay, and his ongoing distress about his brother's schizophrenia. Sacks suggests that his ambivalence toward his brother was the deciding factor in his leaving England and becoming a neurologist (p. 65). Extended family continues to play an important role, as Sacks's Aunt Len helps him through a depression and believes in him when his parents do not (pp. 163–164). Sacks propels himself forward through emigration, where he begins to acquire a freer lifestyle—riding a motorcycle, weightlifting competitively, and continuing his medical training. This is captured well by the title On the Move, which is taken from a poem by a friend. During this time, Sacks develops an unhealthy dependence on drugs, which is linked to romantic disappointment. He chronicles relationships where there was unrequited love and confusion about negotiating the line between homosocial and homosexual affection, along with some less meaningful encounters. He notes disappointment in not having had a lasting, satisfying relationship, but he does not dwell on this.

Sacks include several passages from old journals in OM. He traces his unfolding commitment to neurology, which takes on momentum when he moves to New York and starts to work at Beth Abraham hospital in the Bronx. He has powerful clinical experiences with backward patients whose lives are transformed through L-dopa, the basis for his book Awakenings (which, of course, was made into a film). He encounters difficulties in his work environment and begins to turn more toward writing. Sacks reports dissatisfaction with the direction of his field, where only the new and recent were recognized, "as if neurology had no history" (p. 102). In contrast, Sacks emphatically notes, "I think in narrative and historical terms" (p. 102).

As Sacks's writing career takes off, he becomes a public figure. In UT, his references are most often to chemists from previous centuries; in OM, Sacks encounters new circles of artist and scientist friends—W. H. Auden, Harold Pinter, Robin Williams, Robert De Niro, Jerome Bruner, Stephen Jay Gould, Gerald Edelman, Temple Grandin, Richard Gregory, and Francis Crick. Yet, he remains solitary and sees this as necessary to sustain his creativity (p. 258). He reiterates his lack of interest in current affairs, "whether political, social or sexual" (p. 237).

A major part of Sacks's life as an adult is his psychoanalysis and, in particular, the relationship he forms with his analyst, Leonard Shengold. As a condition of treatment, Shengold demanded that Sacks give up amphetamines, which he manages to do successfully after a scary manic experience. As Sacks sees it, his abstinence allows the analysis to get under way fully. At first, he is resistant, but then he becames "more open to the analytic process" (p. 146). He articulates this openness in terms of "freedom of communication" that does not defer to "ordinary social intercourse" and that entails tuning in to "what lies beyond consciousness or words" (p. 147). Sacks credits his analysis with unleashing his creativity in his work (p. 276).

It is, no doubt, shocking for anyone outside the psychoanalytic world to fathom how Sacks could have spent almost a half century in treatment. This is less surprising, perhaps, in light of what we learn about Sacks's history, the dual traumas of life at the boarding school and his mother's rejection of his sexual orientation, as well as his (related) adult experience of not finding an enduring, satisfying romantic relationship. Sacks does not disclose much about the content of his analysis. He does note that Shengold and he maintained a formal way of addressing each other as "Doctor." In a private correspondence, Shengold divulged to me that the first time he used Sacks's first name was on the day before he died. Sacks clearly uses his analysis to adopt a reflective stance on his early childhood experience. He identifies with a radio program he heard on evacuees during World War II, where one man describes his unresolved problems with the three B's: "bonding, belonging, and believing" (p. 235). Sacks makes impressive strides in each of these categories by the end of his life.

Whereas *UT* ends on a note of uncertainty, *OM* takes on more pathos as it moves forward. Sacks unsparingly describes grower older, losing sight in one eye, and suffering other ailments. It is especially heartwarming to hear about Sacks finding love in his life at the age of 77 in a relationship with a fellow writer named Billy. Sacks experiences "intense emotionality," a sense of feeling "love, death and transience, inseparably mixed" (p. 380). The unleashing of emotion reveals Sacks's mentalized affectivity, as he has worked through the past and it no longer obstructs his experience of the present or the future. In an exquisite passage, he captures the enormous changes that accompany his experience of falling in love:

> Deep, almost geological changes had to occur; in my case, the habits of a lifetime's solitude, and a sort of implicit selfishness and self-absorption, had to change. New needs, new fears, enter one's life— the need for another, the fear of abandonment. There have to be deep, mutual adaptations. (p. 381)

In finding fulfillment in this relationship, Sacks faces the limits of narcissism and finds happiness in being together with a partner. He describes reading the manuscript of Billy's book *The Anatomist*; he elaborates on their various mutual activities, from concerts to making dinner together.[3]

---

[3] Bill Hayes's (2017) recently published book *Insomniac City* is, among other things, a tribute to their relationship. Hayes observes that Sacks had to learn how to share in their relationship, something he had not done before (p. 163). Overall, he celebrates their love and corroborates Sacks's own experience of the relationship.

Sacks ends *OM* with an affirmation of who he is: "I am a storyteller, for better or worse. I suspect that a feeling for stories, for narrative, is a universal human disposition, going with our powers of language, consciousness of self, and autobiographical memory" (p. 384). It is fitting that Sacks invokes the term "autobiographical memory," as his journey transports us from the past, which, with the help of his analysis, recedes in influence without disappearing and allows him to move forward creatively and personally. Sacks's journey is unique, but his mentalized affectivity allows him to embrace the larger social and cultural aspects of his experience, like the evacuation from London. This is also the saga of a gay man who is free to tell his story because we are more ready to hear it as a culture. Sacks's legacy must remain what it is: that he sacrifices a personal life, for the most part, in order to embark on his trailblazing career as a storytelling scientist. I especially admire Sacks for protesting and refusing to accept the divide between literature and science. (See the Conclusion for my further thoughts on this issue.) His love of his patients is inspiring for anyone who is a clinician.

OM continues to narrate the story begun in *UT*. But no one could fail to appreciate the immense difference in tone. *UT* is forthright, but repressed. *OM* shows our author drifting in purpose, suffering, even in dangerous self-destructive ways, and yet finding his own path through being a clinician and through writing. His writing career takes off contemporaneously with his analysis. Sacks does not provide details about how the analysis helped him.[4] *OM* is a transformative journey, from being rejected by his mother, with whom he had the most important relationship in his life, to becoming able to form a relationship toward the end of his life. This is the limit of what mentalized affectivity can realize—it does not undo the past, but it opens us to a novel, rewarding present and future.

EVEN MORE SACKS

A measure of Sacks's flourishing mentalized affectivity is found in five Op-Ed pieces that he wrote for the *New York Times* prior to his death.[5] Each of these pieces manifests the evolution in Sacks's character that we have witnessed in OM. The Op-Eds appeared have a crescendo effect,

---

[4]It is strange that one of the two reviews of *OM* in the *New York Times* mentions that Sacks was in psychoanalysis briefly in parentheses without discussing it, and the other ignores it completely (Solomon [2015] mentions psychoanalysis, Kakutani [2015] does not).

[5]Publication details for Sacks's *New York Times* Op-Ed pieces can be found in the References.

like the quickening intensity of a heartbeat: July 6, 2013, to February 19, 2015 (17 months later), to June 5, 2015 (4 months later), to July 24, 2015 (6 weeks later), and then to August 14, 2005 (3 weeks later). Sacks died 2 weeks afterward, on August 30, 2015. The Op-Ed pieces are defined by a truthfulness in communication that is rare and moving.

In the first Op-Ed, on July 6, 2013, Sacks celebrates having turned 80 years old. He was infirm, but this was prior to finding out that his cancer had metastasized. He reports being optimistic and enthusiastic, retaining a feeling that life is about to begin. The benefits that he cites of growing older pertain to mentalized affectivity: "the enlargement of mental life and perception" that he experiences, and had been originally described by his father. Even more related to mentalized affectivity is Sacks's suggestion that old age enables us to bind the thoughts and feelings of a lifetime together.

The second Op-Ed, dated February 19, 2015, has a grim announcement: Sacks's ocular cancer has returned and metastasized, and represents a death sentence. He documents his struggles to come to terms with this reality. He invokes David Hume, a favorite philosopher, who wrote a short text on his impending death, confirming his calm and composed character. In contrast, Sacks admits that he is a man of "vehement disposition, with violent enthusiasms, and extreme immoderation in all of my passions." This reminds us of the teacher who warned about Sacks's potential to go too far (and it also complements Sacks's observation in *The Man Who Mistook His Wife for a Hat* about how deficit is the preferred focus for neurologists, rather than excess). However much there is reason to pause over Sacks's motivation to proclaim his death in a daily newspaper, he cannot be accused of trying to make himself look better than he is. Sacks unblinkingly reports on his growing sense of detachment from the world. He acknowledges feeling fear but ultimately emphasizes his sense of gratitude. Gratitude is a highly social emotion that rests less obviously on biological imperatives than on valuing others, or rather, valuing others for what we have received from them. Gratitude fits easily and well with mentalization, and it is appropriate that Sacks concludes this piece by referring to himself as "a thinking animal."

The third Op-Ed appeared a few months later, on June 5, 2015. Sacks is in a playful mood, pondering his experience of mishearing, which occurs with words but not music. Rather than bemoaning the loss of hearing and the ensuing difficulty in communication, Sacks celebrates it. His perspective is consistent with many of his writings, which point to compensation for loss of function from disorders—for example, in an earlier Op-Ed piece from December 31, 2010, on a blind biologist whose tactile giftedness allows him to discern minuscule variations of contour on shells. Sacks provides some amusing examples of mishearing from his own life, like hearing his assistant say she was on her way to "choir practice" rather than to the "chiropractor," or like hearing "Christmas Eve" as a demand to "kiss my feet." Such mishearing represents a kind of choice to loosen the bonds of social constraint. He is not at all embarrassed about mishearing; he relishes it, refusing to adhere or defer to normative expectations about communication. In this piece, he also mentions Freud, valuing his attention to obscure phenomena like slips of the tongue, but also criticizing him for overreaching in his speculation about unconscious motivation and for retreating from considering neural mechanisms. Although Sacks was happy to valorize the impact of psychoanalysis on his life, he had reservations about the theory.

The fourth Op-Ed piece came out just 6 weeks later, on July 24, 2015. Sacks is in a reflective mood—recalling his love of the periodic table, and how turning to understand nature was the way he had coped with his trauma at boarding school. He uses the night sky as a kind of Rorschach test. He reports feeling better after treatment but then suffering a decline. Sacks fancifully mentions the element bismuth, the 83rd metal on the periodic table, signifying hope to live beyond 82 years old, and then plutonium, the 84th metal, registering doubt that he would live until then. As an extraordinary example of mentalized affectivity, he also time travels backward, mentioning beryllium, the fourth element, which brings him back to his childhood.

Sacks's final Op-Ed piece was published on August 14, 2015, just 2 weeks before his death, on August 30, 2015. He offers a meditation on the Sabbath, an impending sign of his destiny, but also the perfect subject for mentalized affectivity. Recall that in *UT*, Sacks traces his distance from religion to his separation from his mother during his boarding school experience. He informs us of his "raging atheism" and also his lukewarm response to Zionism (Sacks spent time on a kibbutz as a young man). In *OM*, when he tells us about his mother's reaction to learning that he was gay, he mentions that his mother was influenced by the antigay passage from Leviticus. In this final Op-Ed piece, Sacks focuses on his withdrawal from religion because of its bigotry and rigidity, which had influenced his mother. The need to distance himself from his mother drove Sacks away from Judaism, but here new thoughts begin to stir.

Sacks introduces us to a member of his extended family, Robert John Aumann, who is observant, and notes that he would have turned down the Nobel Prize he was awarded if it were presented on the Sabbath. Furthermore, Sacks reports a visit to Israel, in which both his partner, Billy, and he are heartily welcomed by Aumann. So, the association between religion and homophobia is interrupted, and it opens the way for him to recall a positive memory of his mother making gefilte fish.

Mentalized affectivity is at work in Sacks's reworking of past experience, with the emergence of a different kind of memory of his mother, and a different kind of experience with Judaism. It does not seem that Sacks is tempted to return to Judaism per se, rather that he appreciates that religion is the repository of some wisdom in building the cycle of rest/death into the frame of life. I cried when I read this piece about the Sabbath, as it beautifully invokes the abiding presence of our internal objects and shows that their meaning and influence can be shaped through mentalized affectivity.

MENTALIZED AFFECTIVITY VIGNETTES

In this final section, I shall introduce some examples of mentalized affectivity in the clinical domain. To be clear, mentalized affectivity is not a by-product of psychotherapy; patients come in with varying degrees of it prior to commencing therapy. However, in my experience, no patient who has improved through psychotherapy has failed to increase his or her capacity for mentalized affectivity. It is possible, though not common, that a patient might increase his or her capacity for mentalized affectivity but not improve in psychotherapy. Call it the Hamlet problem: such patients love to mentalize, but not much changes in their lives. This is not necessarily a case of pseudomentalization, where the quality of mentalization is poor and defensive; rather, it may be an example of immersion in thinking that simply did not generate action. Generally speaking, though, it is fair to assume that mentalized affectivity will produce changes not just in thought, but in life.

Working on mentalized affectivity is not necessarily easy or quick. However, not everyone needs to spend half a century in treatment, as Sacks, did; and not every patient is as gifted at telling his own story. Yet, my choice to include autobiographical narratives is designed to be exemplary: every human being has a kind of story about his or her life, and psychotherapy is about making the story more explicit. This does not mean that therapy requires the creation of an autobiographical narrative. Therapy is about helping patients feel better about their lives, which can be accomplished in multiple ways.

It is worth clarifying that mentalized affectivity is both retrospective and prospective. It can entail reviewing the past, but it ought to lead us forward. Mentalized affectivity does have a bearing on our quality of life. What this means is a bit complicated, as mentalized affectivity does not banish painful experiences, as much as it can rearrange how they affect us—as we have seen with Sacks's memoirs and his Op-Ed on the Sabbath. Of course, mentalized affectivity cannot prevent new experiences that are negative—accidents or illnesses, or the death of people we love. It should help us cope with negative experiences, though, to be able to put them in perspective and be less overwhelmed by them.

Given that patients come to psychotherapy with differing capacities for mentalized affectivity, we can distinguish among those who begin as low, medium, and high mentalizers. With low mentalizers, therapists might need to move slowly, working on inspiring curiosity and appreciating how emotions provide information that is too valuable to ignore. Therapists should discern where patients might have problems—with identifying, modulating, and/or expressing emotions—and concentrate on building skills in those areas.

Is there such a thing as a patient who cannot learn to mentalize? Realistically, there are patients for whom exploration of the past is disorganizing and disruptive. For such patients, mentalizing must focus on the present, as MBT recommends in treating patients with severe personality disorders. Moreover, low mentalizers, precisely because they start as beginners, sometimes can make incredible strides forward.

There is no question that medium mentalizers can improve through psychotherapy. Their limits are less pronounced, and they can be encouraged to incorporate their past without risk of serious regression. In considering high mentalizers, we might legitimately wonder why they would need to come to therapy, if they are already inclined toward mentalizing their emotions. It is a benefit to come to therapy ready to reap the rewards, but sometimes patients are mentalizing at a level that is not specific enough. So, therapy can help high mentalizers to mentalize more effectively.

What follow are three vignettes, focusing on low (Bernardo), medium (Ava), and high (Carl) mentalizers. I justify these three categories as making sense theoretically and based on research we have done (Greenberg et al., 2017), though clearly more empirical research is needed to support their validity (and indicate whether other categories ought to be considered as well). These vignettes simply convey the potential for psychotherapy to have an impact on mentalized affectivity, and the consequences on the lives of the patients in question.

Bernardo's mentalized affectivity grew over the course of psychotherapy, but he was not someone who, by nature, was curious about his emotions. Recall that he was mandated to come to therapy for continuing anger management in connection with keeping his addictions under control. So, he did not arrive at therapy with an understanding or expectation of what it would be like, and, as I have reported, my impression on meeting him was that it was unlikely he would be interested in pursuing therapy. I was wrong. On reflection, I wonder about my countertransference: Was I afraid of him? Was I afraid I would not be able to help him? Was it his own fear in coming to therapy that was projected into me?

Psychotherapy helped Bernardo to experience emotions besides anger, to be able to modulate and tone down the expression of his emotions, and, more generally, to want to move to have a different life from his family. By taking the lead and wondering how his actions might be perceived by others, I was able to help Bernardo appreciate how he escalated conflicts automatically. Meaningful change occurred when he could see that his reactions were a choice on his part, and that his reflexive reactions were not serving him well.

Bernardo was not comfortable recalling the past, and for a long time I did not push him to do so. His memories from childhood were mainly of episodes of violence—between his father and him, but between his parents as well. In fact, it is worth noting that Bernardo's family culture, going back several generations, was violent and antisocial. Ethnically, Bernardo's family was Mediterranean, but he did not have a strong identification with this culture, preferring the self-image of being a regular American guy. There was not much space in his family life accorded to recollecting the past when Bernardo was growing up, or even as a young adult.

Over time, I realized that it was disorganizing for Bernardo to reflect on the past. So, the bulk of our work focused on the present, and how he might handle situations more constructively. This often meant picking up the pieces after unfortunate incidents in which he lost his composure. Through our work, he got better at restraining himself, and he also experienced a wider palette of emotions. The emotion of sadness was new for him, at least being able to acknowledge it comfortably, and it became the dominant way for him to grapple with the past. Bernardo was never interested in creating an autobiographical narrative about his life. His capacity for mentalized affectivity improved, assessed by a shift from my pushing him to mentalize to his taking this up by himself; but it was limited by the fact that his past felt like a dead weight. He came to therapy with an autobiographical narrative somewhat along the lines of "it was bad, it got worse, but now, at least, at some moments, it seems better." There is no question, though, that Bernardo benefited from therapy, and it must remain unknown, if he had continued, what the ceiling for mentalized affectivity might look like.

The vignette of medium mentalized affectivity concerns Ava, the patient I discussed in Chapter 2 on modulating emotions. Ava had trouble modulating her emotions, and both under- and overreacted in different situations. She had been sexually abused as a child and had attempted to work on this in a previous therapy. That therapy helped her begin to appreciate the implications of the abuse on her current life, but it also led her to confront her mother, with disastrous results. Ava's mother told her if she ever brought up the accusation against the neighborhood boy again, she would be banned from visiting home. Ava was appalled at this, and it helped us to clarify her mother's difficulties as a parent when she was growing up. Ava stopped therapy for a number of years, and when she returned to begin with me, she was determined to make sense of the experience of abuse, which continued to bother her. She likened her state of mind to being unable to digest food, feeling it sitting in your stomach, and suffering on account of it. Her stories of the abuse were horrible, and went considerably beyond bullying, as she was the object of the boy's sadism. (Years later, Ava had heard that the boy apparently ended up in a job that might well allow for his sadism to be practiced.)

Ava was reluctant but willing to explore the past. She suggested that she did not require an empathic response, so I listened and only occasionally made sure to communicate my distress at what she had endured. My stance helped provide confirmation that she had been victimized, which, sadly, her mother refused her. Toward the end of our work, Ava produced a series of new memories of her mother, where she could see how overburdened her mother was dealing with mental illness in the family. This image of her mother contrasted with the image of her mother as protecting the abuser and supporting social propriety over caring about her own daughter. The memories of the abuse did not disappear because the patient added to her perspective on her mother. The new perspective counterbalanced her negative feelings about her mother, but it did not lead to their disappearance. The autobiographical narrative we forged together incorporated the abuse, but Ava's pain began to recede and became less intrusive. So, Ava was less burdened by the past, and she became more grounded in the present. Ava was not, however, open in terms of imagining the future.

The progress Ava made in exploring her own history helped her feel better, and it also had a dramatic effect on her family life, where her emotional vicissitudes smoothed out, and her family noticed and valued the change. She was able to respond more effectively at work, too, getting appropriately angry rather than minimizing her feelings. Ava started therapy with a fair degree of mentalized affectivity. She responded to psychotherapy well, as it allowed her to "digest" the painful history that she knew was there. Ava had a busy career and family life, and stopped therapy after seeing the positive results. Her life was haunted by the abuse only at those times when she thought about it, a significant change. I would guess that there might be a time when she will want to resume psychotherapy.

My vignette concerning a high mentalizer is about a patient who was not discussed in prior chapters of this book. Carl was in his early

30s when he came to see me. His mother had bipolar disorder and was manic and psychotic at times during his early life. His mother oscillated between being loving and attentive and being frightening, intimidating, and out of touch with reality. Carl's parents divorced when he was 8 years old; his father encouraged visits but never set up his apartment so that the patient could sleep over comfortably. Carl was born in a war-torn Eastern European country, where both of his parents had grown up. His maternal grandfather was a military man, proud and unapologetic about having a right-wing past. The family on his father's side were mostly leftists. Both parents came to the United States to escape the never-ending internecine battles in their native country.

As a young man, Carl had tried therapy, and had enjoyed it until a disagreement with his therapist led to the end of the relationship. Carl was mild-mannered and cooperative with me, and I wondered what had gone wrong in the previous treatment. When Carl was a young man, he had volunteered to be sent to his native country, then at war, to be a teacher. He survived some frightening experiences and was curious to make sense retrospectively of the state of mind that put him in such jeopardy. For the first 3 years of psychotherapy, Carl talked and I listened. It seemed to startle him when I interrupted with questions or interpretations. It dawned on me that he needed me to remain neutral—ironic in light of the extent to which neutrality is often portrayed as withholding. My voice seemed to invoke his mother, who was unpredictable and could be loving or completely and dangerously in her own head. Even when I imagined I was being gentle and empathetic, it would easily make him feel attacked and become more defensive, more inclined to crawl back into his shell. His vigilance would be reactivated, and he would become tense and mumble his thoughts. Carl was able to move forward if I stayed in the distance, so I chose not to push him to acknowledge me as a person. We were both somewhat cautious and formal with each other.

Carl led the way in exploring the past—he spent time thinking about his choices in light of his history and was curious to understand more about himself. Carl linked his mother's unreliability to his choice to overexpose himself to danger when he was a young man. He was not experienced in being flexibly self-protective, in adjusting depending on how things unfolded. We also worked on how his youthful overexposure had led him to his current career, which was a direct result of his earlier history but no longer satisfying. Carl made the arduous choice of going back to school and training for a new career. He had dated throughout our work together but finally met a woman, also with an Eastern European background (but from a different nation), with whom he fell in love. Carl put a hiatus on therapy without really ending it. At present, he is working in his new career and married to the woman he met, and they now have three children. I see his improvement in mentalizing mostly in the specifics of the memories he recalled and in the complex autobiographical narrative that he created and I followed (this is one form of co-construction). The autobiographical narrative that Carl came to therapy with understandably focused on his relationship with his mother but became more complex through our work. For example, Carl started to have new, positive memories of playing sports with his father and feeling less disappointed with him postdivorce. His autobiographical story was differentiated, and he was able to use it going forward as a guide in his life.

In comparing these three examples of mentalized affectivity, we begin with their different aptitudes, ranging from low to medium to high. Bernardo became a better mentalizer through the work, although he never embraced the notion of an autobiographical narrative. Ava's mentalizing focused on her abuse, so the challenge of developing an autobiographical narrative involved finding a place for that experience but leaving room for her to be formed through other experiences. Ava chose to focus on improving her relationship with her family, which, given her family of origin, seemed beyond the realm of possibility. Carl came into therapy as a natural in mentalized affectivity. However, he had not yet put together connections between his past (placing himself in danger as a young man) and his more distant past (dealing with a mother who at times was attuned and at other times bizarre and completely inappropriate). It was gratifying as a therapist to see how Carl moved from being rigid in his self-understanding to being flexible. Moreover, he sought out a new career in which he would be able to be magnanimous to others.

The higher the patient's capacity for mentalized affectivity, the more likely it is that he or she will invest in forging an autobiographical narrative. This is not to say that ending therapy without an autobiographical narrative must be regarded as failure; on the contrary, as with Bernardo, the treatment might be successful. The investment in forging an autobiographical narrative is a creative project. Thus, we should not expect everyone to embrace it. As a therapist, I feel obliged to encourage my patients to focus on an autobiographical narrative, keeping in mind that all of them come in with one, so we are really addressing how to render the narrative more complex and substantive. Oliver Sacks offers a wonderful example of creating an autobiographical narrative: it sparkles with his own voice, and it communicates an inspiring, joyous, and highly social spirit to readers.

I would not generalize and say it is preferable to work with high mentalizers because the distance they need to travel is shorter. It can be enormously gratifying to work with low mentalizers, precisely because there is so much to be gained. If a patient exhibits little or no interest in mentalizing, the therapist needs to be prepared to lead the way. You cannot get anywhere without establishing a basic sense of curiosity about emotions. Also, it certainly can happen that the patient's mentalized affectivity does not improve through psychotherapy. Interruptions and failures happen in all approaches, and mine is certainly no exception. Mentalized affectivity does not bestow magical self-knowledge, but it does help people feel better equipped to deal with whatever happens in their lives.

 CHAPTER 6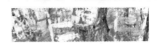

Mentalized Affectivity, Therapeutic Action, and the Communication Paradigm

To discover truth about the patient is always discovering
it with him and for him as well as for ourselves and
about ourselves. And it is discovering truth between each
other, as the truth of human beings is revealed in their
interrelatedness.
— HANS W. LOEWALD, "Psychoanalytic Theory
and the Psychoanalytic Process" (1970)

Mentalized affectivity offers a way to know, use, and communicate emotions that requires engagement with one's history, that is, autobiographical memory. There are many ways to deal with emotions in psychotherapy, and without being specific about this, we risk grappling with emotions in a superficial way. Psychotherapy, if it matters, must transcend immediate relief; it ought to offer patients something that is enduring. In this chapter, I address how mentalized affectivity fosters *therapeutic action,* both during and after psychotherapy, and I make the argument that mentalized affectivity serves to affirm truthfulness, which ties epistemic trust, epistemic vigilance, and communication together. I also venture some thoughts on psychotherapy as an institution within our culture, based on the communication paradigm.

What do I mean by "therapeutic action"? As Lear (2003) proposes, therapeutic action is like an X in algebra, designating both whatever it is that the analyst does by which the patient gets better and whatever

actions can be determined as helping that change occur (p. 31). Therapeutic action, therefore, has a broad-ranging, indeterminate quality concerning the impact of the work on the patient. Lear succinctly places
the accent on the ongoing nature of this process: "Analysis has a termination, therapeutic action does not" (p. 33). The term "therapeutic
action" came into the literature with Loewald's famous essay of the same
title (1960) heralding an era of change in American psychoanalysis to
incorporate objects relations with ego psychology Although it took time
for Loewald's concept to be adopted in psychoanalysis, by now it has
become widely embraced. (see Moscovitz, 2014, for details concerning
its reception). I have chosen to use the term because it represents a crucial turn in the direction of appreciating the role of the relationship in
describing what makes treatment work. Loewald remains bound to the
paradigm of insight but sees insight as occurring through the relationship. As he sees it, the relationship is one of love and bound by truth. I
return to focus on truthfulness in the last section of this chapter, as it is
at the heart of my account of therapeutic action.

In this chapter, I argue that mentalized affectivity provides the best
explanation of what makes therapeutic action work. Mentalized affectivity is the capacity that helps us know what is meaningful to us, strive
toward happiness, and weather whatever happens to us in the course of
life. It contributes to the lessening of symptoms, but this is not its primary aim. Let us keep squarely in mind that feeling less bad differs from
feeling well. Mentalized affectivity means embracing life as a radically
unique, individual journey, but one that does not suffer the conceit of
transcending sociality. Mentalized affectivity urges us toward the pursuit of a creative life, but not one that grants us the freedom to deny reality. It is a project of self-definition that acknowledges the value of being
open to how others define us. Ultimately, mentalized affectivity serves
to facilitate communication, which ought to move us toward the fruits
of life and help us to avoid its agonies. This is a never-ending effort, as
long we are alive, through monitoring where we are in the present in
relation to where we have been in the past and where we would like to
go in the future.

ALL GOOD THERAPISTS MENTALIZE

Although mentalizing can have multifarious objects (beliefs, values,
etc.), working on emotions—identifying, modulating, and expressing
them—is an activity of prime importance in psychotherapy. It is difficult to imagine that any psychotherapy orientation would have no
investment in mentalizing about emotions, although this has different

connotations in different theories. Cognitive-behavioral therapy develops cognitive appraisal as the mechanism of working on our emotions. Mindfulness emphasizes the observation and acceptance of our emotions. Both of these approaches, though, tend to be ambiguous about the role of the self. Dialectical behavior therapy incorporates transformation and change but, like emotion-focused therapy, grants the therapist a powerful didactic role.

Mentalized affectivity can be adjusted to accommodate nonpsychoanalytic psychotherapeutic orientations. It adheres to mentalization theory in supporting the growth of the capacity to mentalize, and an appreciation that epistemic trust and epistemic vigilance are required in order for mentalizing to thrive. If epistemic trust is turned off, it is unlikely that one will be curious about emotions, one's own or others. For example, Knox (2016) claims that abuse can produce epistemic mistrust, wherein therapists' interventions can be experienced as repetitions of the abuse. As I discussed in Chapter 4, MBT, the evidence-based version of mentalization theory, was created as a treatment for severe personality disorders, although it is in the process of branching out to become a treatment for various other kinds of disorders.

As a specific treatment, MBT traces its development from attachment theory, so there is an emphasis on insecure or disorganized attachment as the source of mentalization deficits. MBT aims to elicit from patients how they are experiencing their therapists and, most importantly, to put into words and explain why they feel the way they do. MBT values working in the present as a way to ensure that the emotions are alive, and Fonagy (1999) has expressed skepticism about the usefulness of exploring the past. It makes good sense to be wary of open exploration of the past for patients with severe personality disorders, like those who are typically seen in MBT. In Chapter 5, I gave the example of Bernardo, for whom exploration of the past was disorganizing. Furthermore, exploration of the past, if spearheaded by the therapist, carries the danger of biasing the patient toward being compliant with the expectations that come from another, or of backfiring completely.

But what about patients who want and need to talk about the past? That is, patients who know that things have happened in their lives that weigh on them, which might be vague, dormant but present, or which pop up acutely in unbidden ways? The past is with us whether we like it or not, and the belief that the past does not impinge on the present and the future is naive and interferes with living a fully meaningful life. Insofar as mentalized affectivity involves autobiographical memory, we need to help patients elicit the past as manageable, as real, but also as *not* governing what has not yet happened.

The recent emphasis in mentalization theory on epistemic trust is heartening, as it affirms the importance of the relationship in making therapy effective. Applied to mentalized affectivity, epistemic trust means that there is a collaboration between patient and therapist so the patient feels able to benefit from communication with the therapist, and ultimately with others as well. Beyond helping patients communicate, psychotherapy can result in a better organization of the patient's emotional memories. A patient ought to feel that painful memories are less haunting (or haunting in a less pervasive way), and the work ought to promote space for positive emotions and, overall, a full range of emotions. Moreover, following the suggestion of Mahr and Csibra (2017), we can understand episodic memory as an effort toward veridicality, not just recall of past events; thus, psychotherapy can help patients weigh and assess the meaning of past experience.

As I have stated in Chapter 5, though, the aim of psychotherapy is not strictly to create an autobiographical narrative, and creating a narrative is more likely to be part of a psychodynamic therapy than a CBT therapy. However, regardless of psychotherapeutic orientation, it is important to respect that creating a narrative will be more of a priority for some patients more than for others. Although the memories ought to come from the patient, they require a response from the therapist, who helps the patient make and transform the meaning of his or her experience. The intersubjective aspect, involving both therapist and patient, serves to mitigate confirmation bias, where there is the danger of a patient reinforcing his or her beliefs without reexamining them.

Naturally, patients rarely seek out psychotherapy in order to become better mentalizers. They come because, presumably, they do not feel so good and would like to feel better. It is questionable, in fact, whether and to what degree patients have to be introduced to these concepts. To be clear, mentalizing helps patients to feel better, but patients don't need to understand what mentalization is.

The therapist's perspective is different. Practicing as a therapist *must* include mentalizing , although there is also room for other things, like support. Cognitive-behavioral therapists mentalize; psychoanalysts mentalize. Mentalization-based therapists take this a step further: they mentalize and share their mentalizing with their patients, and push their patients to mentalize as well. At the risk of sounding polemical, I do not believe that I have ever helped a patient without mentalizing about and to the patient. Moreover, like a mentalization-based therapist, I mentalize in order to stimulate the patient to mentalize—to mentalize about me, about himself or herself, or about us as a dyad.

Mentalizing about emotions is the path to knowing what one feels and to action; it adds fine-tuning, or what Barrett (2106) has termed "granularity," to our experience. Granularity connotes seeing things in focus, in detail, and with perspicacity; it represents the polar opposite state to aporetic emotions.

The capacity to mentalize is useful in multiple ways. It can be invoked as a way to solve problems, or just to face up to our feelings, for better or worse. It can be deployed retrospectively, to make sense of something that has already happened; or prospectively, to anticipate what is likely to occur in the future. Mentalized affectivity, of course, is no insurance that life will be wonderful or that one's traumas will vanish in the air. It can provide solace, though, in the face of life's slings and arrows.

Mentalizing maximizes the potential for psychotherapy to be successful. Initially, the therapist mentalizes as a spur for the patient to mentalize. It is likely, but not an absolute rule, for the therapist to take the lead in this regard. Debbané and colleagues (2016) emphasize that psychoeducation about the opacity of mental states is a helpful intervention with adolescents at risk for psychosis. At the same time, therapists should be wary of mentalizing if it is met with passive acceptance by the patient.

The stance of not knowing is particularly important for any mentalizing approach to therapy. Ideally, what happens is that the therapist and the patient learn to mentalize together, to work collaboratively. In fact, joint mentalizing is the basis of the patient's having a new and fulfilling experience through the therapeutic relationship. Joint mentalizing does not mean the therapist and patient will always agree; having space for tolerating differences is perfectly consistent with mentalizing. But, in sum, psychotherapy, by definition, is a place where mentalizing is not done alone.

Fonagy and Allison (2014) stress that mentalizing is not the aim of therapy. The objective must be for the patient to feel better. However, as I argued in Chapter 4, mentalizing is not merely a means to an end. Mentalizing provides its own reward, so feeling well is not simply a consequence or outcome of mentalizing. And yet, mentalizing has limits—it would be grotesque to imagine that, in life, we always must be seeking to mentalize. Mentalizing properly ought to be in the background during some activities, like dancing or making love. Ironically put, mentalizing can help us to stop mentalizing when it is not necessary or helpful.

Mentalizing well means knowing when and when not to mentalize. From an evolutionary perspective, mentalizing is a costly activity, taking us offline in order to fathom something that is ambiguous, hopefully resulting in our participating more meaningfully in social life.

It can take a long time to mentalize emotions well. We fail at it, we fail even when we practice, and no one does it easily. Still, cultivating mentalized affectivity lies at the heart of the enterprise of psychotherapy. It leads to the experience of change and progress, insofar as those are possible.

THE DYNAMIC BETWEEN THE PATIENT AND THE THERAPIST

Mentalizing can be about the self or about the other. Optimally, mentalizing is conceived in terms of being able to use others in the way one thinks about oneself. What seems crucial is being open to consider how one's effort at self-understanding can be augmented by input from outside of oneself. This can be especially challenging when it comes to revealing personal life experiences.

Mentalized affectivity is the path to promoting the patient's agency, so it entails redrawing boundaries between self and others. At the same time, because of its welcoming attitude to others' perspectives, mentalized affectivity is not just about individuation. We lack words to describe being open to influence from others that differ from the language of dependence. Indeed, in Western culture, there is a fear of compromising autonomy (the literal meaning of "autonomy" is being a law unto oneself) through connection to others. As a concept, mentalized affectivity fits well with Blatt's (2008) twofold focus on the coordinates of autonomy and relatedness in personality. The communication paradigm affirms the depths of our sociality, which means psychotherapy must address patients as social beings, not just individual beings.

In a recent article, Fonagy and colleagues (2015) highlight the importance of communication in the evolution of our species, detailing the deleterious implications of lack of epistemic trust and the potential to revive it through psychotherapy. Fonagy and colleagues make the argument that at the heart of psychotherapy is "the recovery of the capacity for social information exchange" (p. 598), and they add the challenging point that change is more likely to occur in the patient's social environment than in therapy itself (p. 599). Their focus is on severe personality disorder, and they specifically argue that borderline personality disorder ought to be regarded as a failure of communication. Without epistemic trust, they argue, communication is not possible, and the patient cannot thrive as a social being.

I concur that without epistemic trust, therapy is not likely to be successful. Yet, epistemic trust yields to epistemic vigilance, as this is where the dynamics of self and other emerge and come to the forefront of the therapeutic relationship. Epistemic vigilance helps patients move beyond insight and incorporate practice into the work. With epistemic trust, the patient has the more passive role of learning from the therapist.

In contrast, with epistemic vigilance, the patient assumes an active role, discerning differences in the input from others, including the therapist. For example, epistemic vigilance can lead a patient to question what a therapist has said, and to do so without the specter of the loss of epistemic trust. A further consequence of epistemic vigilance is that it leaves more room for the patient to address to what extent he or she wants to conform to social and cultural expectations.

The role of the therapist has a complexity that, at first glance, might not be apparent. Psychoanalytic therapists tend to be more comfortable portraying the relationship between patients and therapists in terms of closeness: the quality of the relationship being equated with strong, positive feelings. However, the relationship has a more general social aspect as well—one that serves as an important reminder that the patient does not really know the therapist, because the therapist is relatively restrained about what he or she reveals. Correspondingly, patients will bring different strengths and weaknesses concerning their ability to maintain relationships. For example, a high-functioning person with narcissistic personality disorder might be well adjusted in the arena of general, social relationships, but quite impoverished and unsuccessful in the arena of close, intimate relationships.

In drawing a distinction between close, personal, intimate relationships and general, social relationships, keep in mind that a continuum exists: relationships fall somewhere in between these two categories. Relating to others in a general way means according respect to what one does not know about the other and assuming that the other is not able to see us as we see ourselves. Such relationships are no less relevant in psychotherapy than close, personal ones are. A legitimate aim of psychotherapy is to enable a person to be able to communicate effectively across a range of social relationships from the most general to the most personal.

EPISTEMIC CIRCUMSPECTION

Mentalized affectivity thrives where there is familiarity and knowledge between people. Building a therapeutic relationship (or alliance) is critical for creating the conditions for work to be done. If epistemic trust is lacking, as Fonagy notes, the patient might not be open to receive communication from the therapist. The work in such cases, at least initially, is to foster a kind of earned trust. This clears the way, so that transference and countertransference material can emerge and be processed. Epistemic trust, applied to the clinical realm, does not require a patient's passively accepting whatever the therapist says, or even that the role of the therapist is as an instructor. It suggests only that the patient is open and receptive to the therapist as someone who is trying to help.

Ideally, what happens once epistemic trust is kindled (or rekindled) is that epistemic vigilance can be fostered. Vigilance suggests a more active role for the patient. The connotation of watchfulness is appropriate, but more in the sense of observing and weighing than of being suspicious and reactive. Although epistemic vigilance is already a widely accepted term, "epistemic circumspection" is more descriptive, conveying a less negative and more neutral take: caution, rather than suspicion; the ability to look around, rather than being reactive. Both vigilance and circumspection go beyond sensing danger, and entail comparison and judgment. They are overlapping terms; thus, I am imagining that through the acquisition of experience, vigilance can evolve into circumspection.

In Chapter 4, I focused on epistemic vigilance as a developmental concept that manifests itself around 3–4 years old. However, it is relevant clinically, bearing a relation to the already familiar but not well-defined notion of "reality testing." Epistemic vigilance plays a "filtering role," according to Sperber and colleagues (2010), allowing us to discriminate information that can be trusted from information that cannot be. In other words, epistemic vigilance characteristically emerges when toddlers start to interact more outside of the family, with peers at preschool and on the playground. Children learn that not all information can be trusted; indeed, that blind trust would be a risky and counterproductive automatic strategy. Thus, epistemic vigilance exists in order to help us know what to believe, and what to question.

Epistemic vigilance marks the reality that deception is a factor in communication, requiring us to be able to discern the intentions of others, and to fathom our own intentions as well. Sperber and colleagues (2010) point to the connection between epistemic vigilance and false beliefs, given that children at 3–4 years old recognize that others can be dishonest and incompetent. Without epistemic trust or epistemic vigilance, patients might experience therapists precisely along these lines: as deceitfully intending to mislead them or as wholly unable to contribute anything valuable.

If we suppose that epistemic trust is established or rekindled, how can therapists help patients work on epistemic vigilance? First, therapists can inquire whether patients can articulate reasons for their beliefs or their skepticism of (others') beliefs. Therapists regularly do this, and enjoining patients to spell out their thoughts is often revelatory. Second, therapists can actively encourage patients to compare and evaluate beliefs, promoting on a personal level what is related to the activity of "critical thinking." If a patient is trying to decide whether a person and the beliefs he or she espouses are reliable, a therapist might wonder if the person or beliefs remind the patient of anything (including, for example, actual history with that person). Third, therapists can model epistemic vigilance by being open to reevaluating their views and welcoming patients to express disagreement. Fourth, and perhaps most importantly, as Mahr and Csibra (2017) maintain, episodic memory contributes to epistemic vigilance, so therapists can spur vigilance by wondering about or invoking memories that might illuminate the present circumstance. Recall that episodic memory, in Mahr and Csibra's account, is about justification, not just recall. Clearly, therefore, all three of these points dovetail, as articulating reasons, comparing and evaluating beliefs, and justifying episodic memories converge as communication.

TRUTHFULNESS OR THE LOVE OF TRUTH

Therapeutic action can be realized through mentalized affectivity, which I understand as part of communication. Communication is based on the building blocks of epistemic trust and epistemic vigilance (and circumspection), which flower into complex mind reading, deriving from episodic memory. But a necessary element for mentalized affectivity to succeed is truthfulness—both the therapist's and the patient's love of truth. Truthfulness, in my account, provides both the motivation to engage in the project of mentalized affectivity and a guarantee that the results have substance and value. At first glance, my proposal about truthfulness might seem farfetched, as we can presume that patients seeking psychotherapy want to feel better, not to become philosophers. However, truthfulness is implied in epistemic trust, insofar as we are crediting others with possessing it, in epistemic vigilance, insofar as we are assuming the burden of discerning truthfulness from its imposters, and in autobiographical memory, insofar as it relies on episodic memory, which we have ascertained entails the search for justification.

Interest in truth seems to have receded in our field with the increased emphasis on the therapeutic relationship as paramount. One exception worth noting is a recent special issue of *Psychoanalytic Quarterly* (Volume 5, Issue 2, 2016), which focuses on truth. With few exceptions, the essays convey a wariness of endorsing truth, along with concerns about abandoning it entirely.

Loewald, a psychoanalyst with a background in philosophy as a student of Heidegger, was unusual in making truth central to his understanding of the value of psychoanalysis. He is such an extraordinary thinker precisely because he holds on to the side of being a psychoanalyst that is like being a scientist, yet is unabashed in acknowledging the value of love (Loewald, 1960). When Loewald introduces the notion of love and respect, he is referring to the analyst's genuine emotional engagement with the patient, and he analogizes the relationship between analyst and patient to the relationship between parent and child to explicate this. Loewald repeatedly focuses on communication through the language of the analyst, saying less about communication from the patient. Although I have some reservations about the parent–child analogy and find Loewald's commitment to objectivity to be undertheorized, his valuable main thrust is to affirm the abiding value of the love of truth. Loewald (1970) specifically invokes the phrase "love of truth," which he avers "cannot be isolated from the passion for truth to ourselves and truth in human relationships" (p. 297). The epigram at the head of this chapter supports the notion of truth as intersubjectively constituted.[1]

The distinction between truth and truthfulness is a central concern of philosopher Bernard Williams (2002). Williams follows Nietzsche in arguing that we ought to abandon absolute truth as a fantasy that meant something to philosophers in the past, but that doing so would *not* have to entail giving up truthfulness as an ideal. Truthfulness, as Bernard Williams defines it, relies on two things: accuracy and sincerity. I suspect most therapists would find it easier to accept sincerity compared to accuracy.

Sincerity overlaps with authenticity, a well-established concept in the literature on psychotherapy.[2] A therapist who is insincere or inauthentic is not likely to engender trust. Still, there are difficult questions lurking here. Being sincere, being authentic, and being committed to truthfulness should not be equated with compulsive truth telling. Therapists need some latitude not to divulge what they really think where they imagine that is what is genuinely in the best interests of patients. Truthfulness inescapably entails judgment.

Accuracy is a controversial aspect of truthfulness, as it would have to rely on confirming claims as right, and there are hard questions about how this happens. Can accuracy be guaranteed by the therapist's knowledge? Must the patient concur with the therapist? Alternatively, we might consider whether truth emerges from the intersubjective, collaborative

---

[1] Loewald tries to steer us between the Scylla and Charybdis of absolute truth and relativism. I do not pursue Loewald's ideas further in this context, as they would require more of a detour into both Nietzsche and Heidegger, and they deserve to be pursued as a topic unto itself.

[2] Allen (2016) has focused independently on Williams's work on truthfulness in relation to mentalizing, as part of his larger argument in support of how philosophical ethics illuminates clinical work. Allen's view is influenced by Rogers, and he is more optimistic than I am about the potential of therapists to be transparent.

work of both the therapist and patient. We have evolved beyond imagining that accuracy is primarily a function of the therapist's brilliant insight, and we are more willing to see the role of a therapist as encouraging and corroborating (or not) a patient's self-understanding. Perhaps, accuracy is consistent with the value of being self-correcting; so it need not imply a final, ultimate standpoint.

Prioritizing truthfulness over truth is a way to acknowledge that we aspire to the truth, even if we cannot possess it. The rejection of truth espoused by some postmodernist advocates is a kind of posturing aimed to overthrow the hubris of absolute truth. But human beings want and seek truth, regardless of whether we can attain it in its absolute form. As valuing animals, we make comparisons among our beliefs, discerning some as better than others. Confirmation often eludes us, but is it really intelligible giving up the love of truth? Reflecting on our feelings must involve pondering what might be true, what seems true, and especially what seems to be truer.

Psychotherapy is not exactly a linear path toward truth. The love of truth entails only that we embrace its pursuit. We no longer need to feel the burden of absoluteness—instantiated, for example, in ideas like being "well analyzed." However, the wish to know what is true, and to communicate accordingly, remains the most exciting and defining part of our work.

The love of truth underlies belief in our work as therapists. No patient leaves a treatment that is successful without an enhanced experience of valuing truth. We cannot give up the search for truth, even if we acknowledge the many pervasive ways that we deceive ourselves. If patients do not arrive loving truth, ideally, they leave with it (increasing the odds that the experience will endure) and, if they leave without it, it is unfortunate.

Psychoanalysts have defended numerous positions regarding truth and truthfulness and their place in the clinical endeavor. Spence (1982, 1983) introduced the notion of narrative truth, which, as Eagle (1984) argues, depends on persuasion more than veridicality. Several of the articles in the special issue of *Psychoanalytic Quarterly* mentioned previously defend post-Bionian views: truth as aesthetic (Civitarese, 2016) and truth as emergent (Levine, 2016), both of which challenge the potential to provide evidence in support of truth once we face up to the unavoidable gap between thoughts and words. An interesting recent perspective (and overview of psychoanalytic views) is found in Yadlin-Gadot (2017), who argues that truth is linked to subjective and relational needs, and that "multiple epistemologies and multiple truths" are inescapable. All of these views may be understood as falling under the umbrella of a hermeneutic perspective, given their suspicion of understanding truth as objective and certain. Yet, all of them wish to avoid the specter of relativism.

I have hermeneutic sympathies, but I would locate my position as distinct from the debates of the 1970s, which construed hermeneutics and science as an either/or choice. Affirming the value of a hermeneutic perspective does not have to mean being dismissive of science (Strenger, 2013)—a position I spell out further in Chapter 7 and in the Conclusion. There will always be translation problems in moving from the subjective to the objective (Laplanche, 1989), but this does not absolve us from thinking carefully about what constitutes justification in the subjective realm.[3]

In considering the matter of justification, I would like to sketch out three paths to subjective truth in psychotherapy: accretion, secretion, and excretion. Accretion represents the possibility of accumulating knowledge by adding layers over time—not as sexy as aperçu or insight, but very much a part of psychoanalytic work. The etymology of "accretion" lies in the idea of increasing or adding growth. This happens in therapy through repetition and through looking at the same phenomena from different angles, for example, through episodic memory, which helps us experience or relive deeply felt emotions. Accretion is not a linear process, but one more closely tied to Green's (1999) notion of negation, a Hegelian-influenced concept in which we move forward when we face up to the limits of what we believed to be true and build from there.

Secretion has to do with segregating and elaborating, and is akin to the leaking out of secrets. Despite the similar sound, "secretion" has a different etymology from "accretion," suggesting separating things out. Secretion occurs in unbidden ways and can be thought about as overlapping with enactments, especially ones that reveal something that becomes critical in the mutual understanding of patient and therapist. Excretion is a variation of secretion, where something is dumped out or disposed of, rather than processed and rendered useful. Excretion is related to discharge etymologically; thus, we might think of this term as cathartic—like ridding ourselves of traumatic aspects of memories and excessive self-criticism.

Accretion, secretion, and excretion can operate in relation to each other in different ways. For example, secretion might become part of accretion, and excretion can happen where secretion might be more beneficial. In principle, these three phenomenological categories are healthy and adaptive ways to manifest the pursuit of truth. They do not imply objectivity, certainty, or finality. They do suggest the experience of moving forward, going in the right direction, along with being open to revising one's beliefs. I propose these ideas in the spirit of adding specificity

---

[3]Hanley (2009) refers to accumulating evidence in describing the notion of truth.

to related ideas that have been put forth about subjective truth, like "emotional consensuality" (Civitarese, 2016), "emergent truth" (Levine, 2016), or "vitalization" (Allison & Fonagy, 2016). Allison and Fonagy's (2016) contribution is particularly relevant, as his argument affirms the idea of "felt truth" but ultimately connects this to social context and the role of therapy in promoting communication.

Truthfulness and the pursuit of truth support communication, as they are fundamentally different from persuasion. It is not easy, of course, to stand truth, and Ogden (2016) is wise to observe that the love of truth coexists and must struggle against the fear of the truth. To add a further reflection, given the current political climate, truthfulness is becoming more precious as it recedes from public life. Valued in the private sphere of psychotherapy, it provides respite, but perhaps has subversive potential as well.

PSYCHOTHERAPY AND THE COMMUNICATION PARADIGM

As biological beings, we have evolved to rely on communication, and so psychotherapy exists as a way to foster communication, to inspire interest in it, and to restore it in cases where it has been turned off. Psychotherapy can be construed as a liminal realm, a designated space to step away from the culture to work on participating in a more rewarding way. Without epistemic trust, psychotherapy cannot work; with epistemic trust, it is possible to cultivate epistemic vigilance and circumspection and to make full use of social cognition. Mentalized affectivity ensures the quality of communication by cultivating truthfulness.

The communication paradigm promotes helping patients benefit from and contribute to the social realm. Too casually, we assume that psychotherapy pertains only to the individual qua individual. Yet, there are many questions that go along with this new way of thinking about therapy. Is there a shift implied here about the role of the therapist as an advocate of sociality? How does the meaning of sociality change according to the social location and identity of the patient? There is also no reason to assume that sociality is static and unchanging, so shifts and turns in social trends must affect both therapist and patient.

Ultimately, the communication paradigm brings evolution to bear on our understanding of psychotherapy. Humans have evolved brains that need to interpret face-to-face interactions in small groups, which over time have become much larger groups (see Harari, 2015). We need to know whom we can trust and believe. The communication paradigm affirms the value of general social cognition as well as more intimate relationships.

Of course, not every culture has produced the need for an institution like psychotherapy. While many cultures have place to redress suffering and perhaps someplace for the pursuit of health, psychotherapy comes into being at a particular moment of time. The flesh and blood of actual history supplements the speculative nature of evolutionary explanations.

Psychotherapy comes into being as part of modernity, where there were massive shifts in population from rural to urban life and large numbers of people found themselves living together without the normativity provided by traditional societies.[4] Urban environments were new social laboratories, creating opportunity and risk. Other factors besides the growth of mass society, urbanization, and immigration include secularization and industrialization. Secularization emerges from the embrace of anthropocentrism during the Enlightenment, when humans articulated the ideal of relying on themselves, specifically the capacity to reason, to guide their lives. Secularization explains why someone who is suffering might not automatically turn to a rabbi, priest, or minister.

Industrialization is important, as it provided real changes (including employment) as well as a predominant sensibility of life moving faster and faster. In particular, technological advances inarguably helped to lighten the burden of everyday life, yet produced new and unexpected consequences, facilitating connection but also intrusions from the external world into the private sphere. Indeed, technology facilitates being in touch, but arguably communicating less (Turkle, 2015).

There is one more crucial factor in considering how modernity created the conditions for psychotherapy—capitalism, which underpins all of the other factors I have introduced. Capitalism ensures that cooperation is infused with competition, beckoning us with dreams of success but inflicting a relentless pace, where the thing that matters most is money. Capitalism creates multiple new antagonisms—class divisions, family strife, and alienation.

So far, I have traced some of the forces that propelled modernity and that might have produced the need for an institution like psychotherapy. The invention of psychoanalysis must be understood as a response to and product of the dislocation wrought by modernity. In the course of its century-long history, psychotherapy has followed the lead

---

[4]See Aron and Starr (2013), Cushman (1995), Summers (2013), and Zaretsky (2005) for similar arguments linking modernity and psychotherapy. Freud's life—born in the east (Moravia), raised and resided in a city (Vienna), studied (Paris), and exiled (London)—embodies the movement of modernity. In characterizing Freud in this way, I do not intend to minimize the importance of his identity as a Jew. The relation between Jews and modernity is a separate but fascinating topic (Cuddihy, 1987; Dekel, 2011, Geller, 2011; Goldberg, 2017; Hess, 2002; Horkheimer & Adorno, 1986).

of the culture in focusing on private life over public or social life (Giddens, 1992; Illouz, 2007). Communication represents the beginning of a paradigm shift, which modifies psychotherapy in a way that reflects the needs of our emerging (global) culture.

The communication paradigm aims to improve social cognition and not to restrict itself to personal life. Along the lines I have suggested previously, we can distinguish the different skills and values that accompany general social relations and more intimate relations. This does not mean there is no overlap: it is easy to imagine how the capacity for mutuality, respect, and equality in personal relations could have an impact on general social relations. Some people might need to work on one or the other area of relationships as a priority in psychotherapy. Valuing social cognition is certainly not intended as a way to discountenance the importance of the intimacy aspect of psychotherapy.

Mentalized affectivity, therefore, does not limit itself to individual history and experience. Being open to the influence of others and being invested in various relationships, as we have seen, inherently belongs to mentalizing. Optimally, mentalized affectivity includes attention to cultural memory, not just personal memory, and how this might impact one's understanding of emotions. Indeed, it is not as if there are separate memory banks for group memories and individual memories. An excellent example of what I mean is found in Sacks's recognition of how his trouble with the three B's (bonding, belonging, and believing) was shared with others who were sent away from their families during their bombing of London in World War II.

There is also no reason to believe that it is *only* the relationship with the therapist that matters in psychotherapy, which is a different argument from one that appreciates the importance of the relationship as part of the process. Nor should we assume that it is only what happens within the consulting room that determines the success of psychotherapy and whether a person has changed. Although psychotherapy is an institution within a particular culture, we should be cautious *not* to overlook that its purpose is to promote reentry into the culture. Psychotherapy is a place where people claim a space for reflection with the hope that they can live more adaptively. People go to psychotherapy desiring to feel better, and there is no way around the fact that this impels us to feel more fully and more honestly, and to value truthfulness.

It is a legitimate aim of psychotherapy to support opposition and resistance to the culture, insofar as that is consistent with the desired agency of the patient.

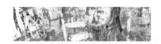 

CHAPTER 7

Mentalized Affectivity
and Contemporary Psychoanalysis

> Seen as a life-political issue, the problem of the emotions
> is not one of retrieving passion, but of developing ethical
> guidelines for the appraisal or justification of conviction.
> The therapist says, "Get in touch with your feelings."
> Yet, in this regard therapy connives with modernity. The
> precept which lies beyond is "evaluate your feelings," and
> such a demand cannot be a matter of psychological rapport
> alone.
>
> —ANTHONY GIDDENS, *The Transformation
> of Intimacy* (1992)

As a concept, mentalized affectivity derives from psychoanalytic ideas but transmutes and rejuvenates them with help from interdisciplinary sources. In this chapter, I bring my understanding of mentalized affectivity into dialogue with contemporary psychoanalytic ideas. By contemporary psychoanalysis, I mean theoretical approaches that do not limit themselves to the (traditional) aim of insight but seek to incorporate aspects of lived experience in the dynamic between analyst and patient. More specifically, I illustrate how object relations and relational theory provide challenges for mentalized affectivity to address. In picking up the story midway through, I am bypassing Freud, not because his views are passé, but because they merit consideration in their own right.[1] My

---

[1] For example, see Jurist (2006) on Freud's complex view of the relation between art and emotions.

ultimate aim will be to suggest that construing therapeutic action as mentalized affectivity and incorporating truthfulness and the communication paradigm represent a new, fruitful direction for contemporary psychoanalysis.

PROTO-MENTAL EXPERIENCE AND LIMITS TO MENTALIZED AFFECTIVITY: BION

Given how difficult it can be to cultivate mentalized affectivity, it behooves us to account for stumbling and even failure—why they occur and how to contend with them therapeutically. Bion provides rich insight on this topic. For him (and for Ferro, whose work we discuss later), emotions manifest themselves between analysts and patients in deep, subtle, and elusive ways. Indeed, in all human interaction, there are limits to the possibility of putting emotions into words.

The mind, according to Bion, is strange, both guileful and alien, and not obscuring this is the unique contribution of psychoanalysis. He makes no bones about ceding to, rather than trying to resolve, ambiguity (Bion, 1962a, Introduction, #5). Bion follows Klein in averring that there is a psychotic element in all of us. He adopts Klein's notion of projective identification, rendering it both ubiquitous and normal (which is not to say that it cannot be pathological). In borrowing Klein's distinction between the paranoid–schizoid and depressive positions, he makes the specific claim that they can coexist (Bléandonu, 1994, p. 155). So, for Bion, we can face reality and fail to do so at the same time.

One of Bion's most extreme and controversial moves is to deconstruct our conventional understanding of being asleep and being awake as opposites, asserting that we dream when awake and that our relation to reality is imperiled if we forsake dreaming. Bion (1973) draws attention to how patients' emotions can be "intense and inchoate," using the terms "sub-thalamic" or "para-sympathetic" (also see Bléandonu, 1994, p. 239). Perhaps, most astonishingly, Bion (1962a) maintains that there is no difference between our emotions when asleep or awake (p. 6). Beyond being a challenge to our conventional assumptions, clearly, the plausibility of this idea must be evaluated by research.

Such ideas are meant to provoke, and perhaps propel us to have the kinds of emotional experiences while reading Bion that he tried to inspire in his clinical work with patients. What comes to mind is Adorno's (1974) famous aphorism that "in psycho-analysis nothing is true except the exaggerations" (p. 49). Should Bion be taken seriously? I would begin with observing that. Bion wants us to appreciate that the mind is not what it seems to be, and that the evidence for this can be glimpsed through what he terms "proto-mental experiences," that is, those that are experienced without being understood. Such experiences, which we all possess, are disavowed as too threatening for the mind to acknowledge. Proto-mental experiences are more readily apparent in infants and psychotics, although adults have them as well.

Following Freud, Bion sees thinking as produced in the face of frustration in early life development, although his emphasis is on the issue of whether the frustration can be tolerated.[2] If an infant cannot tolerate being frustrated—like waiting to be fed—he or she flees from feeling overwhelming pain, resulting in the use of excessive projective identification. Bion suggests that the infant is thereby drawn to omniscience, and, in addition, is not able to discern what is true and false, or what is moral and not. The consequences of such internal experiences are acute confused states. In other words, Bion provides one explanation of what I have termed "aporetic emotions."

If the infant is able to tolerate frustration, then thinking can emerge and reality can be recognized. In Bion's seminal article "A Theory of Thinking" (1962b), he describes how thinking arises from thoughts; so, thinking occurs when there is an active thinker. Yet, Bion is hardly defining thinking in terms of rationality; in fact, thinking serves the valuable function of allowing dreaming to thrive.

Keep in mind that the infant's thinking can occur only with the appropriate response of the caregiver. This is what Bion labels "containment." The infant is in danger of being overwhelmed by various stimuli if the so-called "beta elements," or raw sensory material, cannot be transformed into "alpha elements." Alpha elements become the material that is then used in dreams, fostering the agency and health of the infant. In Bion's early work, he uses the term "psychic growth," but in his later work, he is more cautious about using language that implies progress and he opts to use the term "transformation."

Like Winnicott, Bion anticipates the most basic insight of mentalization theory: that being mentalized about leads to the capacity to self-mentalize.[3] Similar to Bion's conception of thinking, mentalizing is a live activity that initially relies on a conducive environment in which the caregiver's reverie takes in and alters the infant's overpowering emotions, rendering them bearable and available to be used. Without the input of the other, it is impossible that thinking would emerge.

---

[2] In tying his account of cognition to the breast, Bion is affirming a questionable proposition that should be abandoned by psychoanalysts, given the wealth of research that documents the wide range of impressive cognitive abilities that infants possess independent from oral satisfaction.

[3] Indeed, in a recent article, Fonagy candidly acknowledges what he owes Bion and refers to "scotomizing our own indebtedness" to him (Fonagy & Allison, 2016).

Bion is an intersubjectivist, however, only in a partial sense. His view of the mind is that proto-mental experiences can never be eradicated, even when we are able to mentalize, and also that we can never be transparently aware of them. Although we are bombarded with projective identification, the mind remains apart from other minds. Bion does not envision shared mutual experiences, the kind that relational thinkers describe (discussed below). In Chapter 2, I argued that modulation of emotions depends on others, and in Chapters 4, 5, and 6, that mentalizing optimally means being open to how others see you in the way you see yourself. Bion sees thinking as enabling us to "learn from experience," but not specifically to "learn from others."

How does Bion envision therapeutic action? First of all, he does not use this term, and in fact he came to be dubious about the supposition that psychoanalysis must have a goal or telos.[4] Central to Bion's vision of psychoanalysis is the notion of encouraging the patient to embrace process over content, and to be able to stay with present experience rather than retreating into memory. Bion's often-quoted recommendation for the analyst to be "without memory or desire" offers a clear position discouraging fishing expeditions into the patient's past. This was influenced by Bion's personal experience: he referred to his first psychoanalyst as "Mr Feel-it-in-the-past," prior to his more rewarding analyses with John Rickman and Melanie Klein (Bléandonu, 1994). Bion's point of view is well articulated in the following: "Psychoanalytic 'observation' is concerned neither with what has happened nor with what is going to happen but with what *is* happening" (1967a, p. 136, original emphasis). In one sense, I understand this appeal of valorizing live, present experience; in another sense, Bion fails to grapple with complex experiences, where what is happening has already happened in the past.

Ogden (2015) argues that what matters most to Bion in invoking the idea of neither memory nor desire is "intuitive thinking." Does this mean that the analyst should simply rely on his or her emotional reactions to the patient? It seems hard to believe that Bion could be so naive as not to recognize the possibility for intuition to be quite mistaken. As Kahneman (2011) has argued, our intuitions bias us to be wrong—meaning that we should be wary of trusting them, not that we ought to discard them. Using terms from the communication paradigm, it is as if epistemic trust means that there is no need for epistemic vigilance.

Bion's late works move to adopt mysticism. He cites various mystics (Meister Eckhart, St. John of the Cross, Isaac Luria, and the Renan mystics) and introduces the letter "O" to symbolize the unknown and the unknowable. Bion distances himself from a dialectical position between

---

[4] Post-Bionians like Ferro concur, although Ferro (Ferro & Civitarese, 2013) actually does use the term "therapeutic action" in his commentary on Stern (2013b).

knowing and not knowing. Perhaps somewhat ironically, he embraces "the depths of ignorance . . . a frame of mind which as nearly as possible is denuded of preconceptions, theories, and so forth" (1976/1994, p. 307). It seems difficult to reconcile Bion's later works with mentalization, even if we make sure to heed the limits of mentalizing.

Nevertheless, Bion's articulation of the realm of proto-mental experience endures as a valuable counterbalance to construing mentalized affectivity too optimistically as a transparent process. There are limits, and there is no easy, direct path from aporetic emotions to mentalized affectivity.

PROTO-EMOTIONS AND THE ALPHABETIZATION OF EMOTIONS: FERRO AND FIELD THEORY

It says something about Bion that his contribution has prospered in psychoanalysis at the same time that it has diminished in the current mental health world. So-called post-Bionians continue to develop it now. One of them is Ferro, who follows Bion but puts the accent more fully on emotions and how to deal with them in treatment. In that sense, he moves the Bionian perspective forward. According to Ferro (2011), Bion's most important contribution is the notion of the waking dream, and he adopts this in recommending that we listen to patients with this sentence in mind: "I had a dream about this patient . . . " (p. 12). Ferro also strongly identifies with Bion's preoccupation with thinking and regards it as crucial to his own point of view (see Ferro & Civitarese, 2013, which focuses on Bion's article on thinking). As he proposes, the purpose of analysis is to develop "instruments for thinking," rather than "insight, the overcoming of splits, repression, or historical reconstruction" (Ferro, 2015, p. 512).

Psychoanalysis is concerned with the inner world, and the shared inner world of patient and analyst, in Ferro's view. Occasionally, he qualifies this point, saying that this is not meant to indicate "no importance to historical or existential reality" (p. 119). Shortly after this passage, though, Ferro (2011) suggests that: "If analysis is at all possible there is, by definition, nothing that can be outside the analytic relationship—or to put it another way, off-field" (p. 141). The explanation for the exclusive emphasis on what happens within the consulting room is that Ferro believes in the all-encompassing importance of "the field."

Field theory, which has its source in the work of the Barangers (French analysts who emigrated to Argentina and Uruguay) from the 1960s, construes psychoanalysis in terms of the bipersonal field that is created by the unconscious fantasies of both patient and analyst. It is intended to widen the terrain of psychoanalysis beyond the analytic relationship or therapeutic alliance. Yet, the field is "co-determined" (Ferro, 2009). Ferro is influenced by specific components of the Barangers' field theory, such as the bastion (the territory that the patient and analyst collude not to focus on) and the second look (where the analyst opens him- or herself to reevaluating the patient). Compared to Bion, Ferro is more of an intersubjectivist, recognizing the role of the analyst in the process, although he construes this in a less radical way than relational theorists (as I shall discuss in the following section).

Narrativity is another major source of influence on Ferro: he is intrigued by the patients' story, and he introduces stories in his work with patients. He proudly enumerates his love of all kinds of stories— detective stories, thrillers, and science fiction. So, the outside world does become imported, even if Ferro is not invested in the implementation of the patients' understanding in their actual lives. Ferro sees stories as metaphors, and this is central to the way he works with patients.

Ferro's love of stories is contagious and almost makes us forget that the quality of stories varies, from predictable to profound. In the context of discussing metaphor, Ferro (2013) stresses the importance of "living metaphors" (p. 138) and juxtaposes "living and dead metaphors" (pp. 137–138). He explicates this distinction in terms of the former as produced through reverie, whereas the latter comes into existence through free association, which is forced and banal. At one point, Ferro mentions the notion of an "apt metaphor (p. 140), but in general he does not help us to discriminate the use of metaphors in narrative in any evaluative sense. Ferro's vignettes occasionally observe that he is unsatisfied with something he said, and he seems open to recycling metaphors. There is no example, however, of a patient reacting to a metaphor introduced by the analyst as unhelpful or wrongheaded.

Ferro's work is valuable and germane here because of his expansion of what Bion called the proto-mental to the realm of proto-emotions, that is, emotions that are experienced without being understood. Proto-emotions give us a language for making sense of and working with some of what I have termed aporetic emotions. For example, in describing the patient "Luigi," Ferro (2011) suggests that his hyperactivity and inability to read his own mental states means that he exists in a "fog that makes every signal, every letter, every alphabet a blur" (p. 114). Unless proto-emotions are experienced, they risk emerging arbitrarily and as symptoms. Ferro provides a link to specific psychopathologies: "Aggregates of compressed proto-emotions form phobias if the strategy deployed is one of avoidance; obsessiveness, if the strategy is control; hypochondria, if the strategy involves confining it to one organ of the body; and so on" (p. 2).

In order to capture what proto-emotions are and how they act upon us, Ferro (2011) turns to metaphorical language. Proto-emotions pour out of us through projective identification; however, they can also come under the mediated influence of defenses. Ferro's language about proto-emotions is revealing in terms of their lack of granularity: "lumps of emotions" (p. 97) and "lava that as yet cannot be 'held' directly" (p. 98). More recently, he invokes the terms "protoemotional blob" (Ferro & Foresti, 2013, p. 374) and "protoemotional magma" (Ferro, 2009, p. 226). Ferro also speaks about proto-emotions as emotions that are reduced in size and meaning: miniature emotions, or what a patient once termed "bonsai emotions" (p. 3).

How is it possible for proto-emotions to be experienced as emotions? Ferro introduces us to the term "alphabetizing proto-emotions" (2011, p. 67), drawing on the Bionian idea of turning alpha elements into beta elements, and affirming that unformed and inchoate emotions are transformed through being contained. In a striking passage, Ferro (2009) articulates this idea further:

> Upstream of the calcified areas of the stories and the history, there is the process of alphabetization of protoemotional states, in which starting from lumps of emotional alexia, we proceed to lumps of dyslexia, and ultimately to the reading, containability, and transformation of emotions that have a name and a status. The field must contract the patient's "illnesses," and it is only once this happens that genuine transformation will be possible. (p. 219)

Alphabetization relies on language, the effort to give an identity to emotions.

In another passage, Ferro (2011) elaborates as follows: "The purpose of the analysis is to progressively add to the patient's set of tools that enable him to recognize, name, manage, and metabolize emotions" (p. 105). In a recent article, Ferro and colleagues make an explicit link between alphabetization and mentalization (Blasi, Zanette, & Ferro, 2017). Insofar as mentalizing has a containing quality, there is a good fit. However, Ferro expresses views that are incommensurate with mentalization theory, dismissing empirical research and infant observation as valuable only in terms of generating metaphors (p. 85).

Ferro endorses Bion's insight that process matters more than structure in psychoanalysis. He reiterates this point many times and notes accurately how it dovetails with Fonagy's mentalization theory (Ferro, 2011, p. 173). Ferro is not as skeptical of memory as Bion—he welcomes stories as a desirable part of analytic work, and stories often recall the past. Ferro acknowledges that he likes to quote from films and literature in talking to patients and in his writing. He also notes the analogy between psychoanalysis and painting, insofar as the work serves to create verbal pictures, or what become "emotional pictograms." Ferro is captivated by using the idea of character as a way to describe the roles played both by patients and analysts in the stories that are created in the field.

Following Bion, Ferro (2011) is committed to the development of the "creative potential of the human being" (p. 50), and he also introduces multiple metaphors to explicate his theoretical and clinical work. Whereas Bion tended to use digestive and sexual metaphors, Ferro introduces gastronomical and cinemagraphic ones. Metaphors do not just facilitate our understanding; they are transformative and ultimately serve to restore the bodily element to the mind (Civitarese & Ferro, 2013). Ferro's metaphors range from the astute (comparing analysis to cooking, with the analyst as chef and the field as an analytic kitchen) to the hilarious (proto-emotions as "freeze-dried food") to the ridiculous (conjuring the risk of mental Chernobyls). Relying on metaphors is evocative, and supports the aspiration of encouraging patients to live more fully and creatively. Yet, Ferro does not linger long enough to ponder that not all metaphors are created equally—not all of them can work well, some must bomb, and some may capture the phenomena only slightly.

Both Bion and Ferro draw our attention to a rudimentary channel of communication of emotions. Emotions exist prior to and apart from being put into words; correspondingly, language alters emotions as it conveys meaning.[5] The notion that there is a rudimentary channel of emotions to which we are denied direct access is a valuable qualification, reminding us that mentalization has limits, and that it operates at the edge of our awareness. Mentalizing shares a speculative element with metaphor and should never be misconstrued as a printout of the depths of our minds. As with mentalized affectivity, metaphors are a way for our emotions and thoughts to mingle freely. As an example, recall Sacks's use of metals as metaphors in *Uncle Tungsten* from Chapter 5.

While the notion of encouraging all patients to live creatively is appealing, it is fair to wonder how to balance it with the necessity of facing reality. For Bion and post-Bionians, this is not a problem, as they imagine that there is a freedom to be claimed in deconstructing the conventional distinction between dreams and reality. Indeed, Ferro suggests that metaphor is the royal road to reality, an evocative but wholly unsupported claim. Certainly, reality is not a monolithic rock, as it fluctuates

---

[5] I would like to stake out an agnostic rather than dogmatic position regarding the relation of proto-emotions and language. How can we know that language must alter or distort proto-emotions? Is it not possible to imagine that, on occasion, language manages to provide a good translation? If we analogize proto-emotions to music, is there no such thing as poetic lyrics that fit the music? It should be clear that by raising these questions, I am not intending to doubt the notion of the dynamic unconscious itself.

and is subject to alteration. Yet, it seems cavalier not to worry about underestimating or forsaking reality.

Mentalized affectivity inspires us to engage reality, that is, to hold on to the ambiguity of not being too deferential or too dismissive of it. The idea that the only thing that matters is psychic reality has outlived its usefulness No doubt, good reasons exist to be wary of defining therapeutic success in terms of concrete changes in the patient's life—like getting married or finding a new job. Still, I find it thrilling when I realize that a patient has translated something from psychotherapy to life outside. Although Ferro alludes to the potential of creating "collective myths" through psychoanalysis, his approach lacks focus on humans in context, and thus transformation ultimately pertains to the patient qua individual, not as a social being. Ferro never addresses how the social, cultural, and political interpenetrate the field. But others have worked on that question, which I discuss under the rubric of "Relational Mentalizing."

RELATIONAL MENTALIZING I:
GREENBERG AND MITCHELL, ARON, AND BENJAMIN

Contemporary mainstream psychoanalysis has remained largely unpolitical and unconcerned with social problems or social justice. An exception is the (American) relational movement, led by analysts who were influenced by the 1960s and have sought to rebel against and restructure the official culture of psychoanalysis. Such relational thinking has made a key contribution to mentalized affectivity and therapeutic action. The first research in this area comprises the work of Greenberg and Mitchell, Aron, and Benjamin. We focus on that first, and then turn to the work of Bromberg and Stern.

The relational movement arrived on the scene as a breath of fresh air. It represented a different mentality from the depiction of psychoanalysis found in Janet Malcolm's *Psychoanalysis: The Impossible Profession* (1981) and *In the Freud Archives* (1984). Not only was relational theory open to sources outside of psychoanalysis, such as feminism and postmodernism, it opened a path away from the stultifying influence of psychoanalytic institutions that were dominated by the medical profession. Within the culture of psychoanalysis, the relational movement stands for resisting authoritarianism and establishing more of a democratic spirit on every level—among colleagues, between candidates and analysts, between supervisors and supervisees, and especially between patients and analysts.

Greenberg and Mitchell's (1983) *Object Relations in Psychoanalysis* is the foundational text of the relational movement, articulating a new paradigm, in sharp contrast to psychoanalytic theories that have a drive structure. Indeed, Greenberg and Mitchell reject any possibility of mediating between the models, specifically discounting the viability of mixed-models thinkers like Mahler, Jacobson, Kernberg, Kohut, and Loewald. For Greenberg and Mitchell, the emphasis placed on knowledge in the drive model is impossible to reconcile with the emphasis on the relationship in the relational model.

Arguably, the most important contribution that has emerged from the relational model is in the realm of technique, which has implications for therapeutic action. Greenberg and Mitchell (1983) introduce a new role for the analyst as a participant in the process, not someone who is outside or above it. As Mitchell (1988) argues, "If the analytic situation is not regarded as one subjectivity and one objectivity, or one subjectivity and one facilitating environment, but *two subjectivities*—the participation in and inquiry into this interpersonal dialectic becomes a central focus of the work" (p. 38, quoted in Aron, 1991, p. 44). The point is not merely that the analyst possesses subjectivity as the patient does, but that the analyst can use his or her subjectivity in order to make therapy more effective.

Aron (1992) developed the notion that the analyst's subjectivity can be fruitfully brought to bear in treatment. He advocates a spirit of "co-participation" between analyst and patient, a "bipersonal and reciprocal communication process, a mutual meaning-making process" (p. 504). As Aron (1991) sees it, this approach more honestly acknowledges the fact that patients are able to mentalize the analyst, regardless of a neutral stance:

> Patients make use of their observations of their analyst, which are plentiful no matter how anonymous the analysts may attempt to be, to construct a picture of their analyst's character structure. Patients probe, more or less subtly, in an attempt to penetrate the analyst's professional calm and reserve. They do this probing not only because they want to turn the tables on their analyst defensively or angrily but also, like all people, because they want to and need to connect with others, and they want to connect with others where they live emotionally, where they are authentic and fully present, and so they search for information about the other's inner world. An analytic focus on the patient's experience of the analyst's subjectivity opens the door to further explorations of the patient's childhood experiences of the parents' inner world and character structure. Similarly, patients begin to attend to their observations about the characters of others in their lives. (pp. 35–36)

Patients are mentalizing about us whether we are aware of it or not. It is compelling to urge us not to experience a patient's curiosity in a negative way. Yet, I have trouble accepting Aron's generic claim because it overlooks the diversity of responses that patients have to their therapists, which includes intense interest, both positive and negative, but should not exclude vague, ephemeral interest, or even actual indifference. After a break from my private practice due to the death of my mother, it was my most psychotic patient who noticed and overtly expressed that something major must have just happened in my life. Yet, I have also had patients who were not so curious about me, and some who, in being encouraged to voice their thoughts and reactions, warmed to the idea, as well as others who retreated from this. In Chapter 5, I describe a patient, Carl, who had a mother with bipolar disorder. Carl needed distance between us and was averse to the expectation that he would engage with me personally. I have also had the experience of talking more about myself than I typically do with a patient who would have been completely content with a tepid transference, as he had with his prior therapist.

In the context of suggesting that therapists ought to welcome and value patients' reactions to them, Aron tells us, "I assume that the patient may very well have noticed my anger, jealousy, excitement, or whatever before I recognize it in myself" (1991, p. 37). This is revelatory, as it supports the effort of relational analysts to level the playing field between patient and therapist, not just on ideological grounds, but simply because patients, like all others, can observe things about analysts that we fail to observe ourselves. In his recent work, Aron affirms the idea of the analyst's vulnerability, that is, of being capable of mutual vulnerability in his or her relationship with patients, the antidote to the posturing omniscient analyst: "phallic, abstract, rational, autonomous, disembodied, a blank screen, a surgeon" (Aron & Starr, 2013, p. 397). Hiding behind the mantle of a professional identity obscures what we share with patients as fellow human beings. What Aron is saying supports my finding in Chapter 2 that the regulation of emotions often involves others, and my observation in Chapters 5 and 6 that having a therapist mentalizing about you is a spur toward mentalized affectivity.

The analyst who has best articulated the import of mutuality in the relational model is Jessica Benjamin. Mutuality between patient and analyst is modeled on the mutuality found in the infant–caregiver relationship. Benjamin's first book, *The Bonds of Love* (1988), traces this idea from Hegel, where mutual recognition is threatened by the master–slave dialectic, in which competition and violence prevail over cooperation. Recognition involves both shared experience and acceptance of differences between self and other. Winnicott (1965) and Stern (1985) are invoked as the sources for the idea that the mind is interactive, rather than monadic, and both intersubjectively constituted and inherently social.

Benjamin is a complex theorist whose understanding of mutuality has shifted and developed over time (Jurist, 2000). In *The Bonds of Love*, there was appreciation for the deformation of recognition in the master–slave dialectic, but less focus on the fragility of recognition. In *Like Subjects, Love Objects* (1995), Benjamin gives fuller expression to the inevitability of breakdowns, affirming Tronick and Beebe's research with infant–mother dyads that demonstrates continuous disruptions and repairs, and encouraging the relational model to acknowledge creativity and aggression. In her third book, *The Shadow of the Other* (1998), Benajmin goes further in acknowledging obstacles to recognition, observing that omnipotence "is and always has been a central problem for the self" (p. 85). Benjamin takes pains to explicate that her defense of intersubjectivity, or a two-person psychology, is not at the expense of intrapsychic life, or a one-person psychology.

Benjamin's work has moved on to articulate the idea of the third, a new way to characterize mutual recognition in human relationships, especially between patient and analyst. In "Beyond Doer and Done To: An Intersubjective View of Thirdness," Benjamin (2004) sketches the aspiration for mutual recognition in relation to the pernicious but pervasive dynamic of "doer versus done to," that is, where the lure of claiming the status of being a victim prevails over taking responsibility in relationships. The real downside to the doer-versus-done-to dynamic, or what she labels as the "complementary mode," is that it interferes with conflict being "processed, observed, held, mediated or played with" (p. 9). In contrast, the idea of the third means a kind of intersubjective relatedness that is linked to Winnicott's notion of potential or transitional space. The fruition of thirdness is shared experience, but shared experience that does not entail the blurring of individual identities.

Two distinct kinds of thirdness are specified. The first, the One in Third, stems from early life experience: it is energistic, rhythmic, and naturally entails the accommodation of the other. The One in Third corresponds with infant research that has demonstrated skills like turn taking that are crucial in terms of helping the infant not just to feel connected to the other but to learn from the environment and become acculturated. The second, the Third in One, is a moral stance, where one party is willing to be vulnerable (to say "I'll go first," as Benjamin puts it) to help to cultivate reciprocity, but where differentiation from the other is constitutive of the experience. Invoking morality here raise questions, as it is unclear if Benjamin would be comfortable assuming a universal version. Her primary motivation in this essay is to emphasize two different levels of the third: the former is "protosymbolic communication" and the latter is the "symbolic third." Both are necessary, however more weighty the Third in One seems to be.

Benjamin's understanding of therapeutic action depends on the analyst's capacity to be vulnerable, humble, and compassionate, similar to Aron's. Yet, Benjamin amply appreciates that the virtue of the analyst is no assurance that the third will be sustained. The potential regression from thirdness to twoness in the form of doer versus done is perpetual and does not necessarily come from the patient's resistance. (Benjamin is devastatingly astute in discerning how therapists tend to blame patients for impasses in the work.)

The emphasis on mutual shared experience is crucial, as it pushes the mentalization construct in a new, heretofore unacknowledged direction. Mentalizing is not just about the self or about the other, or even about the self, engaged in trying to make use of the other. It can unfold as a mutual process. Although Benjamin does not focus much attention on affects or emotions (which are not referenced in the index of her books), her sensitivity to the power dynamics between self and other illuminate an aspect of mentalized affectivity that resists models in which the therapist instructs the patient on what and how to feel.

From *The Bonds of Love,* Benjamin has incorporated a social and political commitment in her work. Her argument, affirming the infant–caregiver bond, is a feminist battle cry to rebel against construing this bond as inherently maternal. Benjamin specifically forecasts social change as dependent on men embracing childcare and, more broadly, not defining themselves as spectators of domestic life. Furthermore, the master–slave dialectic, which disrupts mutual recognition, is applicable to gender relations. So, there are parallels between recognition on an interpersonal level and a social level. Benjamin's idealism is sustained in her notion of the third, and in her commitment to theory as a form of praxis.

RELATIONAL MENTALIZING II: BROMBERG AND STERN

Two other relational analysts I discuss are Philip Bromberg and Donnel Stern. Bromberg's relational approach has its source in the interpersonal tradition, and he fits the label that Stern (2013a) has described as "interpersonal–relational." Briefly outlined, Bromberg's major premises are (1) that developmental trauma is part of everyone's history (presumably distinguishing between this small t and the capital-T "trauma" associated with the diagnosis PTSD); (2) that dissociation is a normal, even adaptive feature of the mind (although it can be used defensively, that is, pathologically); (3) that the experience of the self as unitary is an illusion, and that the self, in fact, is composed of multiple self-states (or what corresponds to the decentered self); and (4) that our expectation of how the mind works should accept the limits of the possibility of integration in favor of the linking that Bromberg calls "standing in the spaces."

Like other relational analysts, Bromberg embraces intersubjectivity and construes the role of the analyst more actively than classical analysts. He refers to the notion of "affective honesty" by the analyst and welcomes enactments as opportunities. He finds Benjamin's idea about the third appealing, although Benjamin (2013) has articulated a difference between them in terms of the change from dissociation to conflict in Bromberg versus the change from dissociation to recognition in her work. In other words, Bromberg does not go as far as Benjamin in envisioning therapeutic action as transformative. It seems right, too, to see that Bromberg has less at stake in reimagining the role of the analyst, as he is focused on patients' unique, individual self-states.

Bromberg's well-known idea of "standing in the spaces" is captivating. If the self is defined by multiple self-states and dissociation is a normal feature of the mind, how is it possible for connection and communication to emerge across those states? Bromberg (1996) proposes that standing in the spaces is "an internal linking process" of self-states. The idea denotes the capacity to make room for subjective reality that is not readily containable by the self that is experienced as "me" at that moment (p. 274). Bromberg describes the benefit of standing in the spaces as increased tolerance for internal conflict, but also an "increased capacity to experience and resolve intrapsychic conflict" (p. 288).

Bromberg provides a crucial hint about how to construe "standing in the spaces" by associating it with mentalization. While he rejects the idea of ego integration, Bromberg is open to a process that allows us to own up fully to our various mental states. This "owning up" happens, as he sees it, through retrospectively understanding enactments, where dissociated ideas come to be experienced. In his more recent work, Bromberg (2011) focuses on how trauma alters the mind so that it becomes vigilant in anticipating repetition, in his words, a "smoke detector," ready to be set off at any moment. Bromberg conveys hope that working through enactments can help such patients regulate affect states more adaptively.

Bromberg tries to promote therapeutic action by establishing an environment that is safe, but not too safe. He gives us examples of leading the patient with "safe surprises." He uses the language of "perception" to express how patients begin to have new experiences. Bromberg is intrigued by how patients can avail themselves of new ways to process experience. Following Greenberg and Mitchell, Bromberg questions whether psychoanalysis is about acquiring knowledge in and of itself. Out of all relational thinkers, Bromberg has noted his affiliation with mentalization theory. He has written brilliantly and amusingly on the popular film *Analyze This* in a piece he titled "Mentalize This!" (Bromberg, 2008, 2011; also see Jurist, 2016, for a commentary).

Relational thinkers focus on how the relationship between the patient and analyst fosters therapeutic action. All relational thinkers are sensitive to the therapist's own implication in the process and welcome open and honest communication, valorizing moments of mutuality. Surprisingly, relational thinkers have not addressed the subject of emotions as much as one would suppose (see Spezzano, 1993, for an exception). The contribution of relational thinkers is most powerful in terms of fathoming subtle aspects of the dynamic between self and other that define the psychoanalytic process.

Indeed, the relational movement has been exemplary in trying to lead psychoanalysis away from its history of elitism and to reestablish it as a form of therapy "for the people," in Aron's words. Along with Harris, Dimen, Davies, Corbett, Saketopoulou, and others, Benjamin has argued for taking up gender in a way that has been ignored in psychoanalysis. Others, like Holmes, Leary, Altman, and Suchet, have drawn attention to diversity issues. In one sense, the interpersonal side of relational thinking has always been invested in the social and cultural aspects of human beings. In another sense, relational psychoanalysis has broken new ground in taking up pressing issues concerning diversity. Such issues had been marginal in psychoanalysis, and in mentalization theory.

The relational psychoanalyst Donnel Stern (2013b) has specifically focused on how relational psychoanalysis understands therapeutic action. Stern, like Bromberg, is an interpersonalist, and he contrasts this tradition to Kleinians, Bionians, and post-Bionians because of the extreme emphasis they place on unconscious motivation. For Stern, it is the relationship that allows patients to have new experiences and perceptions. He is particularly captivated by unbidden experience, which is based on what he terms "relational freedom." Relational freedom cannot be chosen; it happens to us, so there can be no such thing as a theory of technique. Although Stern is not as political as other relational analysts, the notion of freedom that he introduces strikes me as an intriguing way to differentiate psychoanalysis from other therapeutic approaches. Freedom captures the potential of treatment to help patients feel good, not just less bad.

Therapeutic action, in Stern's account, is produced by relational freedom. Although the evocative term "relational freedom" is never precisely defined, Stern presents a fascinating case discussion in support of his argument. The patient is a man who is a devoted husband and father with a great career who tends to be self-critical, which manifests itself, on occasion, as anger directed to the therapist. While growing up, this patient suffered a traumatic automobile accident, and his awareness of not really experiencing what happened emotionally, and his evolution toward doing so, is at the heart of the case. Stern has an unbidden experience after the patient endures a tough time, and he finds himself saying to the patient that he could have called him. This leads to the patient's own unbidden experience as he becomes emotional and has an outpouring of tears when Stern goes on to suggest that the reaction might have to do with patient's accident. Stern is adamant that he did not make an interpretation, focusing on the comment about calling him, rather than the linking of the patient's past with his current state of mind. Stern views this interaction in terms of new experience and ultimately relational freedom. The analyst felt free enough to speak without having a clear intention, and the patient had a strongly affective response.

Although the patient and analyst have an experience together, it is certainly led by the analyst, rather than being an experience of mutuality. We are privy much more in this example to the analyst's mentalizing than to the patient's. Clearly, the success of the interaction is seen in terms of the analyst's willingness to be involved and to reflect on that involvement. Stern offers profound insight in noting how much we cling to the status quo, and how challenging it can be to open things up in a new direction without knowing where one is going.

This case also highlights how important the patient's autobiographical memory is, which acquires new meaning. The idea of relational freedom seems closely tied to the idea of epistemic trust, since without that history, the analyst might not have taken the risk, and it would be unclear how the patient might respond. The analyst takes a risk in communicating, and the patient reciprocates communication in a way that changes him. Such unbidden communication in this case is successful, although it would stress believability to ignore the potential for an analyst's unbidden communication to be disruptive. We do not hear whether and to what extent this patient's intense emotional experience exercised an influence on his relationships outside of therapy.

Stern, like many other relational analysts, is enamored with the spontaneity of such an encounter, commenting that reflection tends to lag behind. This is true, but it begs the question of whether retrospectively Stern's intervention, while unbidden, might have been based on a primitive level of emotional understanding and exchange of which he was unaware. In other words, there is an important question of whether unbidden meaning "arbitrarily came to me" or whether retrospectively one can come to understand one's motivation as part of an ongoing effort to forge a new story, in this instance, one where the traumatic accident played more of a part. Stern implies that his relationship with the patient was transformed by this moment, but we never really hear about how it changed their work together. I also wonder, for example, whether there was something in the patient's experience that resonated for the analyst personally. I have dwelled on this example because it fits well with mentalized affectivity. The patient ends up with a better sense of his own experience and how it might have been impacting his life.

THE RELATIONSHIP, BUT NOT JUST THE RELATIONSHIP

All of the psychoanalytic perspectives that I have discussed share an emphasis on a shift away from the classical paradigm. They share a trend toward appreciating the role of the analyst not as observing, but as participating in the process. There is also a shift, as Fonagy, Bion, Ferro, Bromberg, and Stern have put it, in terms of a movement away from content to process. I perceive a consensus among them in valuing the idea of the patient having new experiences rather than acquiring knowledge. For relational analysts, it is not just the analyst who is having new experiences; the notion of the third signifies that both patient and analyst are having experiences together. All of the thinkers whom I have discussed hope to inspire the patient to develop new capacities that will be played out, first and foremost, in the dynamic between patient and analyst. I see mentalized affectivity as consistent with this, although it is distinguished by its emphasis on truthfulness. The relationship and truthfulness go hand in hand in that the former provides the conditions for the latter to thrive.

Let us probe the process/content distinction a bit further. I would agree that we ought to give up prepackaged content—focusing only or primarily on Oedipal conflicts, conjuring one-dimensional, reductionist readings of transference, or indulging in the fantasy of forging an accurate reconstruction of what happened in a patient's life. At the same time, what would be the point of having a capacity like mentalizing, if not to generate new content? Consider Stern's clinical example: the relationship highlights the interaction between patient and analyst in which they engage each other in a new (freer?) way. However, the patient's emotional experience also has an implication for his own story—not just that he had had a single traumatic experience but incorporating that as part of who he is. I am not leaning toward defending content over process here. My point is that process and content are connected, and this means that our understanding of therapeutic action must include questions about whether our beliefs are justified, not just whether they are expressed affectively or freely to the analyst to whom there is a connection. However important and necessary the relationship is to the process, it must contribute to the patient's search to find truthful things about him- or herself.

Although the relationship matters, and matters greatly, we should never minimize its strangeness: it is simultaneously like and unlike any other social relationships. Relational thinkers have touted the experience of the third, that is, our potential to experience subjectively something that is not just subjective. The third emerges from working together, but it is not inconsistent with having moments of disruption or with the space for disagreement between patient and analyst. Moreover, all good therapists appreciate the value of a patient telling us that what we said is not quite right or even wrong. In affirming the value of the relationship, though, we need to recognize the disconsolation that is part of giving up the relationship. Of course, patients carry their analyst with them after termination, but they must resume their lives, better equipped to cope, and ideally seeking to forge or improve other relationships.

Let us come back to the theme of narrativity. As I have said, the archaeological project of seeking truth in the past is problematic and risks being out of touch with the motivation people have in seeking help—to feel better, the sooner the better. The whole project of a fishing expedition, in which miraculously one might get lucky, is deeply flawed and inadequate. Yet, I have committed myself to the notion that the practice of psychotherapy cannot avoid the use of narrativity. Few patients come to psychotherapy requesting a therapist's help assembling a narrative about their lives. Yet, people *do* come to psychotherapy with narratives about themselves, so it is helpful to elicit these narratives, which patients might or might not have much awareness about.

Therapeutic action, therefore, is not a journey from not having a story to having a story about oneself. It is a journey that entails experiencing or, more accurately, reexperiencing emotions and working on understanding, refining, and communicating them. Doing this alone is precarious; mentalized affectivity benefits from having responses from another. What is the relation like, we might wonder, between old stories and the new stories? Would it be fair to see the latter as truer than the former?

New stories do not merely help us to feel better—let's say, at the expense of displacing painful memories. New stories emerge through what I have previously described as accretion, secretion, and excretion. This corresponds to the process of "working through," as long as that term emphasizes the currency of emotions. Loewald's (1960) Homeric image of transforming ghosts into ancestors captures how some qualities of the old stories will remain, but they will affect us in a different way. They will be contained within the emerging space of our hope for a healthy sense of agency. Moreover, the so-called new stories will continue to evolve and change over time.

Bion and post-Bionians are attracted to new stories that are creative; if they are invented, they accept that without rancor or regret.

It is harder to say and generalize about where relational thinkers come down beyond the fact that new stories are forged through the collaborative effort of analyst and patient working together. A striking parallel between both Bion and post-Bionians and relational thinkers is their skepticism that science can help us understand and improve our work. Although Civitarese (2016) suggests that psychoanalysis is "amphibious," both artistic and scientific, he understands truth as "aesthetic," that is, as untranslatable into words. Relational thinkers who defend science exist, like Safran (2012), but he is in the minority. In theories that valorize the relationship, there is a commitment to radical uniqueness and the impossibility of replicating what works. Science is often caricatured as positivistic and summarily dismissed.

This skepticism about science represents a fundamental difference from mentalization theory. As discussed above, MBT has been developed by Fonagy to be an evidence-based treatment for severe personality disorders. My focus on mentalized affectivity is being developed as a measure to assess people's relationship to emotions. Yet, my point is not that science and only science is the answer. Throughout this book, I have looked to autobiographical literature to help us understand emotions and the stories people tell about themselves, supplemented with research about autobiographical memory. So, I support a both/and position, and believe it is especially important for psychoanalysis to be open to ideas from outside of itself, regardless of their source. Indeed, I would turn the skeptical tendency of contemporary psychoanalysis against itself: to claim that science cannot comprehend our work is tantamount to being a definite assertion. It suggests that we can know that we cannot know (through science), rather than the even more thoroughgoing radical claim: that we do not know if we can know (through science) or not. So, the most sober conclusion is to claim that science might help us, not that it will or that it cannot.

In conclusion, mentalized affectivity is a theoretical construct that is being developed through research. The hypothesis that I have proposed—that mentalized affectivity is the path to therapeutic action—has not been tested. At present, the appeal of the construct is how it might accommodate a variety of contemporary psychoanalytic perspectives. In particular, it must account for the post-Bionian notion of proto-emotional states that can be alphabetized and the relational emphasis on mutual mentalizing. The idea of mentalized affectivity adds something to these perspectives in offering a detailed portrait of the multiple ways that emotions are experienced, especially through the lens of autobiographical memory, the embrace of truthfulness, and the communication paradigm.

Conclusion

> Literature and science are creative realms with closely
> related aims. Working in neuroscience labs, teaching
> literature, and writing novels, I have come to see literature
> and science as alternate, equally valid systems for building
> knowledge about human minds. Each realm of learning has
> its strengths and weaknesses, but each creates riches in its
> drive toward understanding.
> —LAURA OTIS, *Rethinking Thought* (2015)

This study of emotions focuses on the varied and fluctuating ways that emotions manifest themselves in human lives. In this book, I have utilized diverse sources to cover as much about our lived experience of emotions as possible—research findings, autobiographical memoirs, and clinical material. Using autobiographical memoirs especially of highly creative individuals like Sarah Silverman (Chapter 1), Tracy Smith (Chapter 2), Ingmar Bergman (Chapter 3), and Oliver Sacks (Chapter 5)—allows us to glimpse how emotions are understood in the course of a life. Using clinical material introduces emotional suffering, where people have sought out help to have a better relationship to their emotions. Given that in three out of four of the memoirs, the authors refer to mental health issues and contact with mental health professionals, caution must be used not to assume that autobiographical writers fit neatly in the achingly vague category of the normal.[1] Given that in the clinical

---

[1] Although Bergman reports having a breakdown and being hospitalized in his memoir, he also claims in an interview with Alan Riding (2007, p. 189) that he was never in therapy.

vignettes, patients have sought help for their problems, they are a step ahead of others who might have problems but have yet to, or will never, seek help.

All of us experience emotional confusion and emotional suffering. What ought to interest us most is what to do with that experience, not just alleviating our bad feelings, but being able to feel fully using our emotions. Using our emotions means being able to identify, modulate, and express them; ultimately, mentalized affectivity is the term that captures our capacity to understand our feelings through our own unique history and memory. Mentalized affectivity provides a means to make sense of whatever happens in one's life and is a guide to be able to handle it well, because it utilizes one's particular knowledge and experience. The journey has taken us from curiosity about knowing emotions (or at least moving beyond aporia and ignorance) to being about to be truthful about our emotions, relying on mentalized affectivity. Mentalized affectivity and truthfulness go hand in hand and are shepherded by the therapist, who as both a general other and an intimate other, can corroborate as well as collaborate with the patient.

TWO CULTURES

As with any study, there are underlying concerns that motivate it and can be made more explicit. In order to do so, I will need to go back to the late 1950s, when C. P. Snow (1959) voiced concern about what he saw as an unfolding and widening divide between the "two cultures" in the West: literary culture and scientific culture. The distinction, while controversial, struck a major chord about an unfolding dilemma, which made discussion across its boundaries difficult and often frustrating. In one sense, the divergence between these two cultures, which Snow described, has only increased further, hardening attitudes and making dialogue seem less possible. In another sense, Snow's concern, which centered on the need to improve education in the sciences, seems outdated, given that scientific culture has become dominant in universities, and the humanities are now facing a crisis of meaning and relevance.

Brockman (1995) has articulated a positive spin on recent developments, invoking the notion of a "third culture," which has emerged from the genre of popular science writing, a phenomenon that is continuing to proliferate. Think of Sacks's oeuvre! Kagan (2009) introduces the notion of "three cultures," including the social sciences as a distinct category and expresses the concern that "big science" has emphasized metrics at the expense of the human subject. However, social science seems to have an uncertain, and possibly lesser status in the academic world—at the college where I teach (the City College of New York), the social sciences division was renamed the Colin Powell School for Civil and Global Leadership (from funds raised by friends of General Powell), which I doubt would have been possible in an earlier era.

Hustvedt (2016) strikes a hopeful tone in imagining "a big beautiful bridge across the chasm," but acknowledges that "at the moment, we have only a make-shift, wobbly walkway," and concluding: "I have noticed more and more travelers ambling across it in both directions" (p. xx). I remain concerned by the dominance of scientific culture within the academy, which seems challenged more by religious fundamentalism than by literary culture. However, I do see my book as a venture across that "wobbly walkway" and am happy to join Hustvedt's bridge-building fantasy

An inescapable, difficult question must be considered: whether the gulf between the two cultures depicted by Snow is being resolved by one culture, that is, scientific, triumphing over the other culture? And another question naturally follows: what might be the consequences of the diminishment of literary culture? Of course, both of these questions become compelling in light of our dependence on technology, which, as Turkle (2015) has observed, imperils our ability to communicate. These are large questions, too large for me to take on directly here. In what follows, I describe some of the implications of the preeminence of science in our culture, beginning with a specific example, closer to home—the field of clinical psychology.

PLURALISM IN CLINICAL PSYCHOLOGY?

It certainly seems fair to say that scientific culture is prevailing in clinical psychology, at least in terms of the preponderant aspiration of the field. This is not exactly a new phenomenon, as it has been present as part of the origins of the field. While psychology never particularly valued literary culture, the ideal of balancing research with clinical wisdom, which was the guiding ideal of the field, has been challenged by a new ideal in which research ought to guide clinical practice. For the record, alternatives models existed, mostly out of favor, which construe scientific methodology broadly and are more receptive to interdisciplinary thinking.

The manifestations of our cultural divide can be glimpsed in the antipathy between researchers and clinicians, which has dramatically increased. For example, Baker, McFall, and Shoham (2008) analogize clinicians to doctors prior to the 20th century, who relied on "intuition and tradition," faith healers whom the public should be wary of. A significant transformation has occurred: away from the scientist practitioner model, which has guided most of the history of clinical psychology, and which espouses a balance between training in science and practice, to the clinical scientist model, where research is supposed to direct practice. McFall, Treat, and Simons (2015) offer a passionate defense of the clinical science model, although they misleadingly suggest that the clinical science model is a reaffirmation of the scientist-practitioner model.

There are pluses and minuses of the clinical science model. In encouraging the field to become more committed to research, it certainly represents a worthy ideal from my point of view. However, it smuggles in assumptions about the need to embrace science as the exclusive path to knowledge that must be brought into the light of day—like the claim that this model ensures cost-effective services (McFall et al., 2015). Encouraging cost-effective services seems benign and practical; at the same time, it is disturbing to ignore where this concern is coming from and how it might weigh uncomfortably with an emphasis on the quality of services and the search for truth. Moreover, the petulant tone of some clinical scientist advocates is born from an anxiety and insecurity about the status of psychotherapy as a science, which has coincided with the not-so-well-known reality that funding for psychotherapy research has become harder to find. This insecurity has gone hand in hand with an increase in posturing and marketing, in contrast to the kind of scientific mentality that deserves to be cherished: modesty and humility (about oneself and one's findings), seriousness (knowing what one does not know), and fallibilism (openness to revising and rethinking what one knows). Here I am verging on dealing with larger issues about science, which should be acknowledged: the expansion of the enterprise of "techno-science" and the corporatization of the university. The identity of clinical psychology has been gripped by science envy, and this has to do with money, power, and prestige, not just love of knowledge.

The aspiration of making psychotherapy more scientific is timely and abidingly worthwhile. In my view (which is based on extensive experience directing a clinical psychology doctoral program and continuing to train clinical psychologists), this entails no justification for neglecting the kind of cultural self-understanding that comes from the humanities. Open-mindedness means being receptive to all sources of knowledge and methodology. This is not a revolutionary point of view; as Woolfolk (2015) amply demonstrates, it is a part of the humanistic tradition in the field. It is consistent, in particular, with what was termed the "scholar-practitioner" model.

There is reason to worry about the direction of the field of clinical psychology, which is promulgated under the latest term of art "health services psychology." Starting in 2017, the Commission on Accreditation of the American Psychological Association has adopted a streamlined approach, differentiating between PhD and PsyD programs rather than the specific models that have existed. In one sense, it is heartening for the field to move away from labels that, as noted, can be deployed polemically. In another sense, I fear that this is a move away from the pluralism of multiple models to two models, accentuating our differences rather than what we share in common. Faculty in PhD programs are defined in terms of doing empirical research, while faculty in PsyD programs can engage in scholarship and/or empirical research.

A pluralistic field is preferable to a field in which science is used as a cudgel to intimidate and silence others. I take seriously the notion that we might learn more from each other by encouraging rather than legislating differences. Why yield to the assumption that valuing science has to entail neglect of other points of view? Acknowledging how much we do not know abets trust and spurs the pursuit of knowledge. Researchers need to be aware of what exceeds their capacity to measure; clinicians would do well not to write off research that fails to capture the subtlety of subjective experience. Scientific posturing, in my opinion, has not produced more respect for clinical psychology. A new strategy, which I have sought to accomplish in this book, embraces a diverse array of sources and interdisciplinary thought.

TRANSLATION

Let us briefly consider clinical psychology in relation to the wider field of mental health. Psychologist researchers have been leaders in creating evidence-based approaches to therapy—with a guiding spirit of developing specific treatments for specific psychopathologies. This is a movement that is moving ahead full steam, as we hear about promising treatments for every imaginable disorder. On the other hand, there has arisen a serious effort to question conventional diagnostic categories, challenging our complacency. Corresponding to the publication of DSM-5 in May 2013, Thomas Insel, former director of the National Institute of Mental Health (NIMH), expressed disappointment that the recently revised volume continued to put too much faith in familiar diagnostic categories and speculated that research funds might be better spent on investigating underlying biological mechanisms of disorders (e.g., neural circuits of fear or working memory). Under Insel's leadership, a new research program, the Research Domain Criteria (RDoC), came into being, which has the potential to revolutionize the field.

The RDoC lay out a promising and comprehensive approach to the search for neuroscientific foundations of mental health and disease. They are based on a matrix that was created by working groups of researchers, which so far has five domains (positive valence systems, negative valence systems, cognitive systems, systems for social processes, and arousal regulatory systems) and multiple levels of how to study these things (genes, molecules, cells, circuits, physiology behavior, self-report, and paradigms). Each of the domains has subcategories (e.g., social processes encompass affiliation, attachment, social communication, perception and understanding of self, and perception and understanding of others) and even sub-subcategories (under perception and understanding of self, there are agency and self-knowledge, and under perception and understanding of others, there are animacy perception, action perception, and understanding mental states). The RDoC represent a broader perspective than the DSM on mental illness. At the same time, they are not a diagnostic system, and only time will tell how varied the research is that they will support. Their strongest commitment is to emerging technology, which is aimed at the neurobiological level. This does not negate interest in psychotherapy, but it suggests that the search for the capacity to examine (and alter) neural networks in real time should become the reigning ideal.[2]

The RDoC represent a spirit of conceptualizing mental disorders as brain disorders, even though they make room for phenomena like social processes. The RDoC hold the promise of putting received wisdom in psychiatry to the test, and perhaps fulfilling the goal of using research to drive practice. Still, many issues will need to be addressed in translating neuroscientific findings to help clinicians aid the suffering human being whom they encounter daily occupying the patient's chair in front of them. In addition to the inevitable, practical issues of translation, there are weighty philosophical issues that are unlikely to vanish in the air. It is reasonable to worry whether the skills of paying close attention to the subjective experience of patients (not to mention to the subjective experience of therapists) will be further diminished in value. Admittedly, clinical work has aspects of both insight and bias, but how could these be teased apart without appreciating the integrity that it takes to do the work well? If we think about the autobiographies and the clinical material we have encountered, it is legitimate to be concerned about the danger of neglecting the importance of sophisticated clinical skills and experience. One initiative that bears notice in this connection is the publication of the second edition of the *Psychodynamic Diagnostic Manual* (Lingiardi & McWilliams, 2017), an attempt to provide a clinically rich and sensitive approach to diagnosis.

---

[2]Insel stepped down as director of the NIMH after 13 years. In his final blog post of October 29, 2015, he makes a plea for humility and for recognizing that we do not yet know much about mental illness. He emphasizes that while the RDoC welcome the study of genes and circuits, they are open to the study of behavior and self-reports. Recently, Insel has acknowledged that the search for biomarkers of mental illness, initiated while he headed NIMH, has failed to contribute to lowering suicide rates or to improving recovery (Rogers, 2017).

SCIENCE, BUT NOT JUST SCIENCE

So far, I have been sketching out a story suggesting that scientific culture is triumphing in the field of clinical psychology and in the wider field of mental health. I think that, for the most part, this is a good thing and will allow these fields to continue to develop and improve. But I am also raising a concern: that it has never been obvious to me why a commitment to science seems to include the denigration of ideas that derive from the humanities. I simply reject the dichotomy that is often assumed. Researchers have cause to be critical of clinicians who are indifferent to their work. However, I also strongly believe that researchers have much to gain from listening well to clinicians and being open to literary culture. Clinical work exposes us to subtleties about emotion, for example, that are ignored at great peril. Indeed, it is a kind of self-deception to fail to notice that psychotherapy reflects, rather than just shaping cultural beliefs and norms, as Woolfolk (2015) and Cushman (1995) have maintained.

In a study of creative thinking in both scientists and artists, Otis (2015) argues that the thinking in these respective fields draws on different strengths. As she proposes:

> Literature and science are creative realms with closely related aims. . . .
> I have come to see literature and science as alternate, equally valid
> systems for building knowledge about human minds. Each realm of
> learning has its strengths and weaknesses, but each creates riches in
> its drive toward understanding. In its quest to reveal the way mental
> worlds work, this book will combine literary and scientific practices.
> Neuroscience and narrative will interact as peers, each able to inspire
> and challenge the other. (p. 13)

Otis's qualitative research interviewing creative scientists and artists challenges our beliefs that are based on distinguishing between visual and verbal skills. She cites research (Kozhenikov, Kosslyn, & Shephard, 2005) that proposes more accurate distinctions among verbal, object, and spatial skills, replacing the older distinction between verbal and visual skills. Many artists have strong object visualization powers, while many scientists have strong spatial visualization powers. However, some of the most successful scientists and artists find ways of building on their natural skill sets, combining their visual and verbal skills. Although Otis focuses on "rethinking thought," the title of her book, and does not deal with emotions, her work has been an inspiration for me in challenging widely accepted assumptions in the study of emotions.

Emotions, the main topic of this book, are the ideal subject to test and address the framing issues I have introduced in the Coda after

Chapter 3. Emotions have become an important object of study across virtually every discipline; they are the substance and marrow of psychotherapy, and crucial for our understanding of mental suffering and wellbeing. The study of emotion provides an excellent testing ground for my perspective that looking to science should not mean looking away from other sources of knowledge. This project encompassed intriguing findings from research as well as subtle, complex variations found in autobiographical narratives and clinical work. At the very least, my ambition has been to question the polarization of the two cultures, and to resist the fervor that renders science the only game in town. By questioning and unsettling the divide between the two cultures, I would like to find new ways to bring them into dialogue.

In this book, I have articulated a way to work with patients on emotions that can be utilized in any psychotherapeutic orientation. All therapists ought to be concerned with whether patients are curious about emotions, and whether they can identify, modulate, and express them. Mentalized affectivity is an outgrowth of mentalization theory, itself a product of psychoanalytic theory. Our experience of emotions necessarily reflects our past history and identity; thus, emotion regulation cannot exist as an abstract category denuded of these factors. Psychoanalytic clinicians are well trained to heed subjective experience and to avoid the language of regulation in a way that distorts our experience and wishes. Would anyone really want to forget about the voice of all unregulated emotions? That strikes me as unrealistic, and so our language of regulation remains in need of refinement in definition and scope.

Psychoanalytic clinicians have also led the way in terms of appreciating the extent to which our emotions are contingent on the emotions of others, including therapists' own emotions. Such recognition has to weigh uncomfortably against the idea that the therapist is the authority in the room. Yet, psychoanalytic clinicians, especially relational analysts, have been far too dubious about science. As I have argued, there is a significant difference between registering doubt and coming prematurely to negative conclusions about the potential of research to help us fathom the practice of psychotherapy. Hopefully, in moving forward, all psychotherapists can embrace the value of helping patients experience their emotions fully, in the apt phrase of Barrett (2014), with granularity. Mentalized affectivity gives us a tool to accomplish this. Ideally, it helps patients to feel and see more clearly—and more truthfully and with a greater commitment to communication. It entails a further process, though, too. Mentalized affectivity is situated in the interstices of who we are and who we might like to become. Psychological health can be a discrete state of mind, but it is also a process or a story that we continue to narrate to ourselves as long as we are alive.

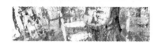 

Mentalized Affectivity Scale

The Mentalized Affectivity Scale (MAS) is a 60-item self-report assessment (see Greenberg et al., 2017) based on previous theorical work of mentalized affectivity (MA; Fonagy et al., 2002; Jurist, 2005, 2008, 2010, 2014), which incorporates mentalization into the process of experiencing emotions. Specifically, the theory suggests that the capacity to mentalize improves emotion regulation, as emotions thereby can be revalued in meaning, not just adjusted upwardly or downwardly. MA is a sophisticated form of emotion regulation that requires the ability to reflect on one's thoughts and feelings and to mentalize about the factors that may influence the experience of emotions, such as childhood experiences or the present situation or context a person is in. Beyond helping us fathom how the past influences the present, MA helps to anticipate future situations.

MA theory proposes three delineated aspects that are part of a concentric process of emotion regulation. The first is *identifying* emotions, which in its most basic form involves labeling emotions but also includes deeper complexities that involve making sense of emotions in the context of one's personal history and exploring the meaning of emotions (e.g., "Why am I feeling this way?"). The second aspect, which follows identifying emotions, is *processing* them. Processing involves modulating/regulating emotions, which includes changing the emotion in some way, such as by duration or intensity. The third aspect, which follows processing emotions, is *expressing* them. Expressing involves communicating one's thoughts and emotions on a spectrum from inwardly to outwardly. A person's prior history influences each aspect of emotion regulation from identifying and processing to expressing. Furthermore, these aspects are tied to a person's sense of agency with emotions—with identifying, there is the dawning of a sense of agency, with processing, there is the actualization of agency, and with expressing, there are the results or manifestations of agency.

PSYCHOMETRICS

The MAS was validated in a nonclinical sample of 2,000 individuals. Principal-components analyses revealed an orthogonal three-component structure underlying MA, which corresponded to the dimensions hypothesized in MA theory: identifying, processing, and expressing. Hierarchical modeling suggested that processing emotions delineates from identifying them, and expressing emotions delineates from processing them. Correlational results showed that these three dimensions were associated with personality traits, well-being, trauma, and psychological disorders (including mood, neurological, and personality disorders). Results also showed how MA scores varied across psychological treatment modalities and years spent in therapy. The scale advances prior research on emotion regulation and mentalization and offers a different perspective from commonly used measures, including the Emotion Regulation Questionnaire (ERQ; Gross & John, 2003), the Difficulties in Emotion Regulation Scale (DERS; Gratz & Roemer, 2004), and the Reflective Function Questionnaire (RFQ; Fonagy et al., 2016).

INSTRUCTIONS FOR USE

The MAS has multiple uses. It can be administered online or via paper and pencil and is useful in both clinical and nonclinical settings. It can be used for social psychological, clinical psychological, psychiatric, big data, genetic, or brain imaging studies. The MAS is free to use for research purposes, but commercial use requires a license. A brief version of the scale is available from the authors upon request. Administration must include a reference or citation for the scale.

Mentalized Affectivity Scale (MAS)

Here are a number of statements about emotions that may or may not apply to you. Please indicate the extent to which you agree or disagree with each statement, using the scale below.

Disagree strongly	Disagree moderately	Disagree a little	Neither agree nor disagree	Agree a little	Agree moderately	Agree strongly
1	2	3	4	5	6	7

1. _____ I often think about how the emotions that I feel stem from earlier life experiences (e.g., family dynamics during childhood).
2. _____ I can express my emotions clearly to others.
3. _____ I am good at understanding other people's complex emotions.
4. _____ I use tools I have learned to help when I am in difficult emotional situations.
5. _____ I can see how prior relationships influence my current emotions.
6. _____ I can still think rationally even if my emotions are complex.
7. _____ I am able to wait to act on my emotions.
8. _____ I put effort into managing my emotions.
9. _____ It is hard for me to talk about my complex emotions.
10. _____ When I am filled with a negative emotion, I know how to handle it.
11. _____ I often know the reasons why I feel the emotions I do.
12. _____ Understanding my emotional experience is an ongoing process.
13. _____ I am often confused about the emotions that I feel.
14. _____ I am able to adjust my emotions to be more precise.
15. _____ It is hard for me to manage my emotions.
16. _____ Knowing about my childhood experiences helps to put my present emotions within a larger context.
17. _____ It is easy for me to notice when I am feeling different emotions at the same time.
18. _____ I often think about my past experiences to help me understand emotions that I feel in the present.
19. _____ I am able to keep my emotions to myself if the timing to express them isn't right.
20. _____ I often keep my emotions inside.

21. _____ I can easily label "basic emotions" (fear, anger, sadness, joy, and surprise) that I feel.
22. _____ I am good at increasing emotions that I want to feel more.
23. _____ I am good at controlling my emotions.
24. _____ When I express my emotions to others, it is usually jumbled.
25. _____ When I am filled with a positive emotion, I know how to keep the feeling going.
26. _____ I am good at controlling emotions that I do not want to feel.
27. _____ I am quick to act on my emotions.
28. _____ It helps me to know the reasons behind why I feel the way that I do.
29. _____ I am aware of recurrent patterns to my emotions.
30. _____ People tell me I am good at expressing my emotions.
31. _____ If I feel something, I prefer not to discuss it with others.
32. _____ It takes me a while to know how I am really feeling.
33. _____ I try to understand the complexity of my emotions.
34. _____ It is important for me to acknowledge my own true feelings.
35. _____ I often figure out where my emotions stem from.
36. _____ If I feel something, I would rather not convey it to others.
37. _____ I often look back at my life history to help inform my current emotional state and situation.
38. _____ I am open to what others say about me to help me know what I am feeling.
39. _____ People get confused when I try to express my emotions.
40. _____ Sometimes it is good to keep my emotions to myself.
41. _____ I am good at distinguishing between different emotions that I feel.
42. _____ I am curious about identifying my emotions.
43. _____ If a feeling makes me feel uncomfortable, I can easily get rid of it.
44. _____ I often know what I feel but choose not to reveal it outwardly.
45. _____ If I feel something, it often comes pouring out of me.
46. _____ I try to put effort into identifying my emotions.
47. _____ I can pinpoint childhood experiences that influence the way that I often think and feel.
48. _____ If I feel something, I will convey it to others.
49. _____ Thinking about other people's emotional experiences helps me to think about my own.
50. _____ I can see how prior relationships influence the relationships that I have now.
51. _____ It is helpful to think about how my emotions stem from family dynamics.
52. _____ I am open to other people's view of me because it helps me to better understand myself.

53. _____ I rarely think about the reasons behind why I am feeling a certain way.

54. _____ It's important to understand the major life events that have had an impact on my behavior.

55. _____ I am not aware of the emotions I'm feeling when in conversation.

56. _____ I am more comfortable "talking around" emotions I am feeling, rather than talking about them directly

57. _____ I am good at identifying my emotions.

58. _____ I can quickly identify my emotions without having to think too much about it.

59. _____ I am able to understand my emotions within the context of my surroundings.

60. _____ I can tell if I am feeling a combination of emotions at the same time.

61. _____ I am interested in learning about why I feel certain emotions more frequently than others.

MAS SCORING

"R" denotes reverse-scored items.

- Identifying: 1, 4, 5, 8, 12, 16, 18, 28, 29, 33, 34, 35, 37, 38, 42, 46, 47, 49, 50, 51, 52, 53R, 54, 60

- Processing: 3, 6, 7, 10, 11, 13R, 14, 15R, 17, 21, 22, 23, 24R, 25, 26, 32R, 39R, 41, 43, 55R, 57, 58, 59

- Expressing: 2, 9R, 19R, 20R, 27, 30, 31R, 36R, 40R, 44R, 45, 48, 56R

For further information, see the Mentalized Affectivity Lab website at *https://mentalizedaffectivitylab.squarespace.com*. Readers who would like to consult with the authors should contact Elliot Jurist (*ejurist5@gmail.com*) or David M. Greenberg (*dmgreenberg87@gmail.com*).

References

Abbass, A. (2016). The emergence of psychodynamic psychotherapy for treatment resistant patients: Intensive short-term dynamic psychotherapy. *Psychodynamic Psychiatry, 44*(2), 245–280.

Abbass, A., & Town, J.M. (2013). Key clinical processes in intensive short-term dynamic psychotherapy. *Psychotherapy, 50*(3), 433–437.

Adorno, T. W. (1974). *Minima moralia: Reflections from damaged life.* London: New Left Books.

Aisenstein, M. (2006). The indissociable unity of psyche and soma: A view from the Paris psychosomatic school. *International Journal of Psychoanalysis, 87,* 667–680.

Aldao, A. (2012). Emotion regulation strategies as transdiagnostic processes: A closer look at the invariance of their form and function. *Revista de Psicopatología y Psicología Clínica, 17*(3), 261–277.

Alexander, F. (1950). *Psychosomatic medicine: Its principles and applications.* New York: Norton.

Allen, J. G. (2016). Should the century-old practice of psychotherapy defer to science and ignore its foundations in two millenia of ethical thought? *Bulletin of the Menninger Clinic, 80*(1), 1–29.

Allen, J. G., Fonagy, P., & Bateman, A. (2008). *Mentalizing in clinical practice.* Washington, DC: American Psychiatric Association Press.

Allison, E., & Fonagy, P. (2016). When is truth relevant? *Psychoanalytic Quarterly, 85*(2), 275–303.

American Psychiatric Association. (2013). *Diagnostic and statistical manual of mental disorders* (5th ed.). Arlington, VA: Author.

Apperly, I., & Butterfill. S. (2009). Do humans have two systems to track beliefs and belief-like states? *Psychological Review, 116*(4), 953–970.

Aron, L. (1991). The patient's experience of the analyst's subjectivity. *Psychoanalytic Dialogues, 1*(1), 29–51.

Aron, L. (1992). Interpretation as expression of the analyst's subjectivity. *Psychoanalytic Dialogues, 2*(4), 475–507.

Aron, L., & Starr, K. (2013). *A psychotherapy for the people: Toward a progressive psychoanalysis.* New York: Routledge/Taylor & Francis.

Bach, T. (2011). Structure-mapping: Directions from simulation to theory. *Philosophical Psychology, 24*(1), 23–51.

Bagby, R., Parker, J. D., & Taylor, G. J. (1994). The twenty-item Toronto Alexithymia Scale–I: Item selection and cross-validation of the factor structure. *Journal of Psychosomatic Research, 38*(1), 23–32.

Baker, T. B., McFall, R. M., & Shoham, V. (2008). Current status and future prospects of clinical psychology: Toward a scientifically principled approach to mental and behavioral health care. *Psychological Science in the Public Interest, 9*(2), 67–103.

Baldwin, J. (2007). The northern Protestant. In R. Shargel (Ed.), *Ingmar Bergman interviews* (pp. 10–20). Jackson: University of Mississippi Press.

Baron-Cohen, S., Tager-Flusberg, H., & Cohen, D. (2000). *Understanding other minds: Perspectives from autism and developmental cognitive neuroscience.* Oxford, UK: Oxford University Press.

Barrett, L. F. (2011). Constructing emotion. *Psihologijske Teme, 20*(3), 359–380.

Barrett, L. F. (2014). The conceptual act theory: A précis. *Emotion Review, 6*(4), 292–297.

Barrett, L. F. (2016, June 3). Are you in despair?: That's good. *New York Times.* Available from *www.nytimes.com/2016/06/05/opinion/sunday/are-you-in-despair-thats-good.html.*

Bateman, A., & Fonagy, P. (1999). Effectiveness of partial hospitalization in the treatment of borderline personality disorder: A randomized controlled trial. *American Journal of Psychiatry, 156*(10), 1563–1569.

Bateman, A., & Fonagy, P. (2001). Treatment of borderline personality disorder with psychoanalytically oriented partial hospitalization: An 18-month follow-up. *American Journal of Psychiatry, 158*(1), 36–42.

Bateman, A., & Fonagy, P. (2006). Mentalizing and borderline personality disorder. In J. G. Allen & P. Fonagy (Eds.), *The handbook of mentalization-based treatment* (pp. 185–200). Hoboken, NJ: Wiley.

Bateman, A., & Fonagy, P. (2008). 8-year follow-up of patients treated for borderline personality disorder: Mentalization-based treatment versus treatment as usual. *American Journal of Psychiatry, 165*(5), 631–638.

Bateman, A. W., & Fonagy, P. (2012). *Handbook of mentalizing in mental health practice.* Arlington, VA: American Psychiatric Publishing.

Bateman, A., & Fonagy, P. (2015). Borderline personality disorder and mood disorders: Mentalizing as a framework for integrated treatment. *Journal of Clinical Psychology, 71*(8), 792–804.

Baumeister, R. F., Zell, A. L., & Tice, D. M. (2007). How emotions facilitate and impair self-regulation. In J. J. Gross (Ed.), *Handbook of emotion regulation* (pp. 408–426). New York: Guilford Press.

Benjamin, J. (1988). *The bonds of love: Psychoanalysis, feminism, and the problem of domination.* New York: Pantheon Books.

Benjamin, J. (1995). *Like subjects, love objects: Essays on recognition and sexual difference.* New Haven, CT: Yale University Press.

Benjamin, J. (1998). *Shadow of the other: Intersubjectivity and gender in psychoanalysis.* Florence, KY: Taylor & Frances/Routledge.

Benjamin, J. (2004). Beyond doer and done to: An intersubjective view of thirdness. *Psychoanalytic Quarterly, 73*(1), 5–46.

Benjamin, J. (2013). Thinking together, differently: Thoughts on Bromberg and intersubjectivity. *Contemporary Psychoanalysis, 49*(3), 356–379.

Ben-Ze'ev, A. (2003). IX. The logic of emotions. *Royal Institute of Philosophy Supplement, 52,* 147–162.

Bergman, I. (1988). *The magic lantern: An autobiography.* New York: Viking.

Berntsen, D., & Rubin, D. C. (2012). Introduction. In D. Berntsen & D. C. Rubin (Eds.), *Understanding autobiographical memory: Theories and approaches* (pp. 1–8). New York: Cambridge University Press.

Bion, W. R. (1962a). *Learning from experience.* London: Heinemann.

Bion, W. R. (1962b). A theory of thinking. *International Journal of Psychoanalysis, 43,* 306–401.

Bion, W. R. (1967a). Author's response to discussions of "Notes on Memory and Desire." In J. Aguayo & B. Malin (Eds.), *Wilfred Bion: Los Angeles seminars and supervision* (pp. 136–138). London: Karnac Books. (Originally appeared as: Notes on memory and desire. *Psychoanalytic Forum, 2,* 279–281.)

Bion, W. R. (1967b). *Second thoughts.* London: William Heinemann.

Bion, W. R. (1973). *Bion's Brazilian lectures 1.* Rio de Janeiro, Brazil: Imago Editora.

Bion, W. R. (1994). Evidence. In W. R. Bion, *Clinical seminars and other works.* London: Karnac Books. (Original work published 1976)

Blasi, V., Zanette, M., & Ferro, A. (2017). Mentalization as alphabetization of the emotions: Oscillation between the opening and closing of possible worlds. *International Forum of Psychoanalysis, 26*(2), 75–84.

Blatt, S. J. (2008). *Polarities of experience: Relatedness and self-definition in personality development, psychopathology, and the therapeutic process.* Washington, DC: American Psychological Association.

Bléandonu, G. (1994). *Wilfred Bion: His life and works 1897–1979.* New York: Free Association Books.

Bluck, S., Alea, N., Habermas, T., & Rubin, D. C. (2005). A tale of three functions: The self-reported uses of autobiographical memory. *Social Cognition, 23*(1), 91–117.

Bogdan, R. J. (1997). *Interpreting minds: The evolution of a practice.* Cambridge, MA: MIT Press.

Bouchard, M., & Lecours, S. (2008). Contemporary approaches to mentalization in the light of Freud's *Project.* In F. N. Busch (Ed.), *Mentalization: Theoretical considerations, research findings, and clinical implications* (pp. 103–129). New York: Analytic Press.

Bouchard, M., Target, M., Lecours, S., Fonagy, P., Tremblay, L., Schachter, A., et al. (2008). Mentalization in adult attachment narratives: Reflective functioning, mental states, and affect elaboration compared. *Psychoanalytic Psychology, 25*(1), 47–66.

Brockman, J. (1995). *The third culture: Beyond the scientific revolution.* New York: Simon & Schuster.

Bromberg, P. M. (1996). Standing in the spaces: The multiplicity of self and the psychoanalytic relationship. *Contemporary Psychoanalysis, 32*(4), 509–535.

Bromberg, P. M. (2008). "Mentalize this!" Dissociation, enactment, and clinical process. In E. L. Jurist, A. Slade, & S. Bergner (Eds.), *Mind to mind: Infant research, neuroscience, and psychoanalysis* (pp. 414–434). New York: Other Press.

Bromberg, P. M. (2011). *The shadow of the tsunami and the growth of the relational mind.* New York: Routledge/Taylor & Francis.

Brooks, D. (2015). *The road to character.* New York: Random House.

Brown, A. D., Kouri, N. A., & Superka, J. E. (2015). Contextualizing traumatic memories: The role of self-identity in the construction of autobiographical memory in posttraumatic stress disorder. In C. Stone & L. Bietti (Eds.), *Contextualizing human memory: An interdisciplinary approach to understanding how individuals and groups remember the past* (pp. 11–22). New York: Routledge/Taylor & Francis.

Brown, K. W., Ryan, R. M., & Creswell, J. D. (2007). Mindfulness: Theoretical foundations and evidence for its salutary effects. *Psychological Inquiry, 18*(4), 211–237.

Burton, C. L., & Bonnano, G. A. (2016). Measuring ability to enhance and suppress emotional expression: The Flexible Regulation of Emotional Expression (FREE) Scale. *Psychological Assessment, 28*(8), 929–941.

Calkins, S. D., & Hill, A. (2007). Caregiver influences on emerging emotion regulation: Biological and environmental transactions in early development. In J. J. Gross (Ed.), *Handbook of emotion regulation* (pp. 229–248). New York: Guilford Press.

Campos, J. J., Thein, S., & Owen, D. (2003). A Darwinian legacy to understanding human infancy: Emotional expressions as behavior regulators. In P. Ekman, J. J. Campos, R. J. Davidson, & F. M. de Waal (Eds.), *Emotions inside out: 130 years after Darwin's "The expression of the emotions in man and animals"* (pp. 110–134). New York: New York Academy of Sciences.

Campos, J. J., Walle, E. A., Dahl, A., & Main, A. (2011). Reconceptualizing emotion regulation. *Emotion Review, 3*(1), 26–35.

Carruthers, P., & Smith, P. K. (1996). *Theories of theories of mind.* Cambridge, UK: Cambridge University Press.

Chambers, R., Gullone, E., & Allen, N. B. (2009). Mindful emotion regulation: An integrative review. *Clinical Psychology Review, 29*(6), 560–572.

Choi-Kain, L. W., & Gunderson, J. G. (2008). Mentalization: Ontogeny, assessment, and application in the treatment of borderline personality disorder. *American Journal of Psychiatry, 165*(9), 1127–1135.

Civitarese, G. (2016) Truth as immediacy and unison. *Psychoanalytic Quarterly, 85*(2), 449–501.

Civitarese, G., & Ferro, A. (2013). Metaphor in analytic field theory. In S. M. Katz (Ed.), *Metaphor and fields: Common ground, common language, and the future of psychoanalysis* (pp. 121–142). New York: Routledge/ Taylor & Francis.

Cole, P. M., Martin, S. E., & Dennis, T. A. (2004). Emotion regulation as a scientific construct: Methodological challenges and directions for child development research. *Child Development, 75*(2), 317–333.

Conway, M. A. (2005). Memory and the self. *Journal of Memory and Language, 53*(4), 594–628.

Conway, M. A. (2009). Episodic memories. *Neuropsychologia, 47*(11), 2305–2313.

Conway, M. A., & Jobson, L. (2012). On the nature of autobiographical memory. In D. Berntsen & D. C. Rubin (Eds.), *Understanding autobiographical memory: Theories and approaches* (pp. 54–69). New York: Cambridge University Press.

Conway, M. A., & Pleydell-Pearce, C. W. (2000). The construction of autobiographical memories in the self-memory system. *Psychological Review, 107*(2), 261–288.

Cuddihy, J. M. (1987). *The ordeal of civility: Freud, Marx, Lévi-Strauss, and the Jewish struggle with modernity.* Boston: Beacon Press.

Cushman, P. (1995). *Constructing the self, constructing America: A cultural history of psychotherapy.* Boston: Da Capo Press.

Damasio, A. R. (1994). The brain binds entities and events by multiregional activation from convergence zones. In H. Gutfreund & G. Toulouse (Eds.), *Biology and computation: A physicist's choice* (pp. 749–758). River Edge, NJ: World Scientific.

Damasio, A. R. (1999). *The feeling of what happens: Body and emotion in the making of consciousness.* New York: Harcourt Brace.

Damasio, A. R. (2010). *Self comes to mind: Constructing the conscious brain.* New York: Random House.

Darwin, C. (1872). *The expression of the emotions in man and animals.* London: John Murray.

Davidson, R. J. (2010). Empirical explorations of mindfulness: Conceptual and methodological conundrums. *Emotion, 10*(1), 8–11.

De Panfilis, C., Ossala, P., Tonna, M., Catania, L., & Marchesi, C. (2015). Finding words for feelings: The relationship between personality disorders and alexithymia. *Personality and Individual Differences, 74*, 285–291.

Debbané, M., Bermiloud, J., Salaminios, G., Solida-Tozzi, A., Armando, M., Fonagy, P., et al. (2016). Mentalization-based treatment in clinical high-risk for psychosis: A rationale and clinical illustration. *Journal of Contemporary Psychotherapy, 46*(4), 217–225.

Dekel, M. (2011). *The universal Jew: Masculinity, modernity, and the Zionist moment.* Evanston, IL: Northwestern University Press.

Diamond, D., Yeomans, F., & Stern, B. L. (2018). *Treating narcissistic pathology: A transference-focused psychotherapy.* New York: Guilford Press.

Eagle, M. N. (1984). Psychoanalysis and "narrative truth": A reply to Spence. *Psychoanalysis and Contemporary Thought, 7*(4), 629–640.

Egyed, K., Király, I., & Gergely, G. (2013). Communicating shared knowledge in infancy. *Psychological Science, 24*(7), 1348–1353.

Ekman, P. (1992). Are there basic emotions? *Psychological Review, 99*(3), 550–553.

Ekman, P. (1996). A lingua franca of facial expressions. *Demos, 10*, 37–38.

Ekman, P. (2003). Darwin, deception, and facial expression. In P. Ekman, J. J. Campos, R. J. Davidson, & F. M. de Waal (Eds.), *Emotions inside out: 130 years after Darwin's "The expression of the emotions in man and animals"* (pp. 205–221). New York: New York Academy of Sciences.

Ekman, P., Campos, J. J., Davidson, R. J., & de Waal, F. M. (Eds.). (2003). *Emotions inside out: 130 years after Darwin's "The expression of the emotions in man and animals."* New York: New York Academy of Sciences.

Ekman, P., & Davidson, R. J. (1994). *The nature of emotion: Fundamental questions.* New York: Oxford University Press.

Ensink, K., & Mayes, L. C. (2010). The development of mentalization in children from a theory of mind perspective. *Psychoanalytic Inquiry, 30*(4), 301–337.

Erisman, S. M., & Roemer, L. (2010). A preliminary investigation of the effects of experimentally induced mindfulness on emotional responding to film clips. *Emotion, 10*(1), 72–82.

Farb, N. S., Anderson, A. K., Mayberg, H., Bean, J., McKeon, D., & Segal, Z. V. (2010). Minding one's emotions: Mindfulness training alters the neural expression of sadness. *Emotion, 10*(1), 25–33.

Feldman, G., Hayes, A., Kumar, S., Greeson, J., & Laurenceau, J. (2007). Mindfulness and emotion regulation: The development and initial validation of the Cognitive and Affective Mindfulness Scale—Revised (CMS-R). *Journal of Psychopathology and Behavioral Assessment, 29*(3), 177–190.

Ferro, A. (2009). Transformations in dreaming and characters in the psychoanalytic field. *International Journal of Psychoanalysis, 90*(2), 209–230.

Ferro, A. (2011). *Avoiding emotions, living emotions.* Hove, UK: Routledge.

Ferro, A. (2015). A response that raises many questions. *Psychoanalytic Inquiry, 35*, 512–525.

Ferro, A., & Civitarese, G. (2013). Analysts in search of an author: Voltaire or Artemisia Gentileschi?: Commentary on "Field theory in psychoanalysis: Part 2. Bionian field theory and contemporary interpersonal/relational psychoanalysis" by Donnel B. Stern. *Psychoanalytic Dialogues, 23*(6), 646–653.

Ferro, A., & Foresti, G. (2013). Bion and thinking. *Psychoanalytic Quarterly, 82*(2), 361–391.

Fertuck, E. A., Mergenthaler, E., Target, M., Levy, K. N., & Clarkin, J. F. (2012). Development and criterion validity of a computerized text analysis measure of reflective functioning. *Psychotherapy Research, 22*(3), 298–305.

Firestein, S. (2012). *Ignorance: How it drives science.* New York: Oxford University Press.

Fivush, R. (2012). Subjective perspective and personal timeline in the development of autobiographical memory. In D. Berntsen & D. C. Rubin (Eds.), *Understanding autobiographical memory: Theories and approaches* (pp. 226–245). New York: Cambridge University Press.

Fonagy, P. (1996). The future of an empirical psychoanalysis. *British Journal of Psychotherapy, 13*(1), 106–118.

Fonagy, P. (1999). Memory and therapeutic action. *International Journal of Psychoanalysis, 80*(2), 215–223.

Fonagy, P. (2006). The mentalization-focused approach to social development. In J. G. Allen & P. Fonagy (Eds.), *The handbook of mentalization-based treatment* (pp. 53–99). Hoboken, NJ: Wiley.

Fonagy, P. (2008a). Early life trauma and the psychogenesis and prevention of violence. In R. Campher (Ed.), *Violence in children: Understanding and helping those who harm* (pp. 33–53). London: Karnac Books.

Fonagy, P. (2008b). The mentalization-focused approach to social development. In F. N. Busch (Ed.), *Mentalization: Theoretical considerations, research findings, and clinical implications* (pp. 3–56). Mahwah, NJ: Analytic Press.

Fonagy, P., & Allison, E. (2014). The role of mentalizing and epistemic trust in the therapeutic relationship. *Psychotherapy, 51*(3), 372–380.

Fonagy, P., & Allison, E. (2016). Psychic reality and the nature of consciousness. *International Journal of Psychoanalysis, 97*(1), 5–24.

Fonagy, P., & Bateman, A. (2010). A brief history of mentalization-based treatment and its roots in psychoanalytic theory and practice. In M. B. Heller & S. Pollet (Eds.), *The work of psychoanalysts in the public health sector* (pp. 156–176). New York: Routledge/Taylor & Francis.

Fonagy, P., Bateman, A. W., & Luyten, P. (2012). Introduction and overview. In A. W. Bateman & P. Fonagy (Eds.), *Handbook of mentalizing in mental health practice* (pp. 3–42). Arlington, VA: American Psychiatric Publishing.

Fonagy, P., & Campbell, C. (2015). Bad blood revisited: Attachment and psychoanalysis. *British Journal of Psychotherapy, 31*(2), 229–250.

Fonagy, P., Gergely, G., Jurist, E. L., & Target, M. (2002). *Affect regulation, mentalization, and the development of the self.* New York: Other Press.

Fonagy, P., Luyten, P., & Allison, E. (2015). Epistemic petrification and the restoration of epistemic trust: A new conceptualization of borderline personality disorder and its psychosocial treatment. *Journal of Personality Disorders, 29*(5), 575–609.

Fonagy, P., Luyten, P., Moulton-Perkins, A., Lee, Y. W., Warren, F., Howard, S., et al. (2016). Development and validation of a self-report measure of mentalizing: The reflective functioning questionnaire. *PLOS ONE, 11*(7), e0158678.

Fonagy, P., & Target, M. (2008). Attachment, trauma, and psychoanalysis: Where psychoanalysis meets neuroscience. In E. Jurist, A. Slade, & S. Bergner (Eds.), *Mind to mind: Infant research, neuroscience and psychoanalysis* (pp. 15–49). New York: Other Press.

Frommer, J. (2013). Contemporary perspectives on psychosomatics in Germany: A commentary on Karen Gubb's paper, "Psychosomatics today:

A review of contemporary theory and practice." *Psychoanalytic Review, 100*(1), 155–165.

Gallagher, S. (2011). Strong interaction and self-agency. *Humana.Mente, 15,* 55–76.

Geller, J. (2011). *The other Jewish question: Identifying the Jew and making sense of modernity.* New York: Fordham University Press.

Gendron, M., Roberson, D., van der Vyver, J. M., & Barrett, L. F. (2014). Perceptions of emotion from facial expressions are not culturally universal: Evidence from a remote culture. *Emotion, 14*(2), 251–262.

George, C., Kaplan, N., & Main, M. (1985). *The Adult Attachment Interview.* Unpublished manuscript, University of California at Berkeley, Berkeley, CA.

Gergely, G. (2007). The social construction of the subjective self: The role of affect-mirroring, markedness, and ostensive communication in self-development. In L. Mayes, P. Fonagy, M. Target, L. Mayes, P. Fonagy, & M. Target (Eds.), *Developmental science and psychoanalysis: Integration and innovation* (pp. 45–88). London: Karnac Books.

Gergely, G. (2013). Ostensive communication and cultural learning: The natural pedagogy hypothesis. In J. Metcalfe & H. S. Terrace (Eds.), *Agency and joint attention* (pp. 139–151). Oxford, UK: Oxford University Press.

Gergely, G., Egyed, K., & Király, I. (2007). On pedagogy. *Developmental Science, 10*(1), 139–146.

Gergely, G., & Jacob, P. (2012). Reasoning about instrumental and communicative agency in human infancy. In F. Xu, T. Kushnir, & J. B. Benson (Eds.), *Advances in child development and behavior: Vol 43. Rational constructivism in cognitive development* (pp. 59–94). San Diego, CA: Elsevier Academic Press.

Gergely, G., & Unoka, Z. (2008). Attachment and mentalization in humans: The development of the affective self. In E. Jurist, A. Slade, & S. Bergner (Eds.), *Mind to mind: Infant research, neuroscience and psychoanalysis* (pp. 50–87). New York: Other Press.

Gergely, G., & Watson, J. S. (1996). The social biofeedback theory of parental affect-mirroring: The development of emotional self-awareness and self-control in infancy. *International Journal of Psychoanalysis, 77*(6), 1181–1212.

Giddens, A. (1992). *The transformation of intimacy: Sexuality, love, and eroticism in modern societies.* Stanford, CA: Stanford University Press.

Goldberg, C. A. (2017). *Modernity and the Jews in Western social thought.* Chicago: University of Chicago Press.

Goldie, P. (2000). *The emotions: A philosophical exploration.* Oxford, UK: Clarendon Press.

Goldman, A. (2006). *Simulating minds: The philosophy, psychology, and neuroscience of mindreading.* Oxford, UK: Oxford University Press.

Goleman, D. (1995). *Emotional intelligence.* New York: Bantam Books.

Gopnik, A. (1993). How we know our minds: The illusion of first-person knowledge of intentionality. *Behavioral and Brain Sciences, 16*(1), 1–14.

Gopnik, A., Capps, L., & Meltzoff, A. N. (2000). *Early theories of mind: What the theory theory can tell us about autism.* Oxford, UK: Oxford University Press.

Gordon, R. M. (1996). "Radical" simulationism. In P. Carruthers & P. K. Smith (Eds.), *Theories of theories of mind* (pp. 11–12). Cambridge, UK: Cambridge University Press.

Gottlieb, R. M. (2013). On our need to move beyond folk medicine: A commentary on Karen Gubb's paper, "Psychosomatics today: A review of contemporary theory and practice." *Psychoanalytic Review, 100*(1), 143–154.

Gratz, K. L., & Roemer, L. (2004). Multidimensional assessment of emotion regulation and dysregulation: Development, factor structure, and initial validation of the difficulties in emotion regulation scale. *Journal of Psychopathology and Behavioral Assessment, 26*(1), 41–54.

Greco, M. (1998). *Illness as a work of thought: A Foucauldian perspective on psychosomatics.* London: Routledge.

Green, A. (1998). Primordial mind and the work of the negative. *International Journal of Psychoanalysis, 79*(Pt. 4), 649–665.

Green, A. (1999). *The work of the negative.* London: Free Association Books.

Green, A., & Weller, A. (2010). Thoughts on the Paris school of psychosomatics. In M. Aisenstein & E. R. de Aisemberg (Eds.), *Psychosomatics today: A psychoanalytic perspective* (pp. 1–45). London: Karnac Books.

Greenberg, D. M., Kolasi, J., Hegsted, C. P., Berkowitz, Y., & Jurist, E. (2017). Mentalized affectivity: A new model and assessment of emotion regulation. *PLOS ONE, 12*(10), e0185264.

Greenberg, J. R., & Mitchell, S. A. (1983). *Object relations in psychoanalytic theory.* Cambridge, MA: Harvard University Press.

Greenberg, L. S. (2015). *Emotion-focused therapy: Coaching clients to work through their feelings* (2nd ed.). Washington, DC: American Psychological Association.

Gregory, A. (2015, November 29). Is it still possible to be a public intellectual? *New York Times,* p. BR27.

Gross, D. M. (2006). *The secret history of emotion: From Aristotle's Rhetoric to modern brain science.* Chicago: University of Chicago Press.

Gross, J. J. (1998). The emerging field of emotion regulation: An integrative view. *Review of General Psychology, 2*(3), 271–299.

Gross, J. J. (2008). Emotion and emotion regulation: Personality processes and individual differences. In O. P. John, R. W. Robins, & L. A. Pervin (Eds.), *Handbook of personality: Theory and research* (pp. 701–724). New York: Guilford Press.

Gross, J. J., & Jazaieri, H. (2014). Emotion, emotion regulation, and psychopathology: An affective science perspective. *Clinical Psychological Science, 2*(4), 387–401.

Gross, J. J., & John, O. P. (2003). Individual differences in two emotion regulation processes: Implications for affect, relationships, and well-being. *Journal of Personality and Social Psychology, 85*(2), 348–362.

Gross, J. J., & Thompson, R. A. (2007). Emotion regulation: Conceptual foundations. In J. J. Gross (Ed.), *Handbook of emotion regulation* (pp. 3–24). New York: Guilford Press.

Grosz, S. (2013). *The examined life: How we lose and find ourselves*. New York: Norton.

Gubb, K. (2013). Psychosomatics today: A review of contemporary theory and practice. *Psychoanalytic Review, 100*(1), 103–142.

Habermas, T. (2015). A model of psychopathological distortions of autobiographical memory narratives: An emotion narrative view. In L. A. Watson & D. Bernsten (Eds.), *Clinical perspectives on autobiographical memory* (pp. 267–290). New York: Cambridge University Press.

Haidt, J. (2001). The emotional dog and its rational tail: A social intuitionist approach to moral judgment. *Psychological Review, 108*(4), 814–834.

Hanly, C. (2009). On truth and clinical psychoanalysis. *International Journal of Psychoanalysis, 90*(2), 363–373.

Harari, Y. N. (2015). *Sapiens: A brief history of humankind*. New York: Harper.

Hayes, B. (2017). *Insomniac city: New York, Oliver, and me*. New York: Bloomsbury.

Hayes, S. C., & Plumb, J. C. (2007). Mindfulness from the bottom up: Providing an inductive framework for understanding mindfulness processes and their application to human suffering. *Psychological Inquiry, 18*(4), 242–248.

Herwig, U., Kaffenberger, T., Jäncke, L., & Brühl, A. B. (2010). Self-related awareness and emotion regulation. *NeuroImage, 50*(2), 734–741.

Hess, J. M. (2002). *Germans, Jews and the claims of modernity*. London: Yale University Press.

Heyes, C. M., & Frith, C. D. (2014). The cultural evolution of mind reading. *Science, 344*, 1–6.

Hofer, M. A. (1990). Early symbiotic processes: Hard evidence from a soft place. In R. A. Glick & S. Bone (Eds.), *Pleasure beyond the pleasure principle* (pp. 55–78). New Haven, CT: Yale University Press.

Hofmann, S. G., & Kashdan, T. B. (2010). The Affective Style Questionnaire: Development and psychometric properties. *Journal of Psychopathology and Behavioral Assessment, 32*(2), 255–263.

Holmes, J. (2015). *Nonsense: The power of not knowing*. New York: Crown.

Horkheimer, M., & Adorno, T. W. (1986). *Dialectic of enlightenment*. London: Verso.

Howe, M. L., & Courage, M. L. (1997). The emergence and early development of autobiographical memory. *Psychological Review, 104*(3), 499–523.

Hustvedt, S. (2016). *A woman looking at men looking at women: Essays on art, sex, and the mind*. New York: Simon & Schuster.

Illouz, E. (2007). *Cold intimacies: The making of emotional capitalism*. Cambridge, UK: Polity.

Illouz, E. (2008). *Saving the modern soul: Therapy, emotions, and the culture of self-help*. Berkeley: University of California Press.

Insel, T. (2015, October 29). Farewell. [Web blog post by former National Institute of Mental Health Director Thomas Insel]. Available from *www.nimh.nih.gov/about/directors/thomas-insel/blog/2015/farewell.shtml*.

Jurist, E. L. (2000). *Beyond Hegel and Nietzsche: Philosophy, culture, and agency*. Cambridge, MA: MIT Press.

Jurist, E. L. (2005). Mentalized affectivity. *Psychoanalytic Psychology, 22,* 426–444.

Jurist, E. L. (2006). Art and emotion in psychoanalysis. *International Journal of Psychoanalysis, 87*(5), 1315–1334.

Jurist, E. L. (2008). Minds and yours: New directions for mentalization theory. In E. Jurist, A. Slade, & S. Bergner (Eds.), *Mind to mind: Infant research, neuroscience and psychoanalysis* (pp. 88–114). New York: Other Press.

Jurist, E. L. (2010). Mentalizing minds. *Psychoanalytic Inquiry, 30*(4), 289–300.

Jurist, E. L. (2014). Whatever happened to the superego?: Loewald and the future of psychoanalysis. *Psychoanalytic Psychology, 31*(4), 489–501.

Jurist, E. L. (2016). Exclamation: Honoring Philip Bromberg. *Division/Review, 15,* 68–69.

Kagan, J. (2009). *The three cultures: Natural sciences, social sciences, and the humanities in the 21st century.* Cambridge, UK: Cambridge University Press.

Kahneman, D. (2011). *Thinking, fast and slow.* New York: Farrar, Straus & Giroux.

Kakutani, M. (2015, April 27). Review: Oliver Sacks looks at his life in "On the move." *New York Times.* Available from *www.nytimes.com/2015/04/28/ books/review-oliver-sacks-looks-at-his-life-in-on-the-move.html.*

Kano, M., & Fukudo, S. (2013). The alexithymic brain: The neural pathways linking alexithymia to physical disorders. *BioPsychoSocial Medicine, 7*(1), 1–9.

Klein, S. B. (2012). The self and science: Is it time for a new approach to the study of human experience? *Current Directions in Psychological Science, 21*(4), 253–257.

Knausgård, K. O. (2013). *My struggle, Book 1* (D. Bartlett, Trans.). New York: Farrar, Straus & Giroux.

Knox, J. (2016). Epistemic mistrust: A crucial aspect of mentalization in people with a history of abuse? *British Journal of Psychotherapy, 32*(2), 226–236.

Koenig, M. A., & Harris, P. L. (2005). The role of social cognition in early trust. *Trends in Cognitive Sciences, 9*(10), 457–459.

Koole, S. L. (2009). The psychology of emotion regulation: An integrative review. *Cognition and Emotion, 23*(1), 4–41.

Kovács, A. M., Teglas, E., & Endress, A. D. (2010). The social sense: Susceptibility to others' beliefs in human infants and adults. *Science, 330,* 1830–1834.

Kozhevnikov, M., Kosslyn, S., & Shephard, J. (2005). Spatial versus object visualizers: A new characterization of visual cognitive style. *Memory and Cognition, 33*(4), 710–726.

Krystal, H. (1988). *Integration and self-healing: Affect, trauma, alexithymia.* Hillsdale, NJ: Analytic Press

Kurzban, R., & Aktipis, C. A. (2007). Modularity and the social mind: Are psychologists too self-ish? *Personality and Social Psychology Review, 11*(2), 131–149.

Laplanche, J. (1989). *New foundations for psychoanalysis*. Oxford, UK: Blackwell.

Lear, J. (2003). *Therapeutic action: An earnest plea for irony*. London: Karnac Books.

Leary, K. (2012). Race as an adaptive challenge: Working with diversity in the clinical consulting room. *Psychoanalytic Psychology, 29*(3), 279–291.

Leary, M. R. (2007). How the self became involved in affective experience: Three sources of self-reflective emotions. In J. L. Tracy, R. W. Robins, & J. P. Tangney (Eds.), *The self-conscious emotions: Theory and research* (pp. 38–52). New York: Guilford Press.

Lecours, S. (1995). *Manuel de cotation de la Grille de l'Élaboration Verbale des Affects (GÉVA)*. Unpublished manuscript, Department of Psychology, Université de Montréal, Montréal, Québec, Canada.

Lee, D., Witte, T., Bardeen, J. Davis, M., & Weathers, F. (2016). A factor analytic evaluation of the Difficulties in Emotion Regulation Scale. *Journal of Clinical Psychology, 72*(9), 933–946.

Legare, C., & Harris, P. (2016). The ontogeny of cultural learning. *Child Development, 87*(3), 633–642.

Levine, H. B. (2016). Psychoanalysis and the problem of truth. *Psychoanalytic Quarterly, 85*(2), 391–409.

Lewis, M. (2011). The origins and uses of self-awareness or the mental representation of me. *Consciousness and Cognition: An International Journal, 20*(1), 120–129.

Lieberman, M. D. (2013). *Social: Why our brains are wired to connect*. New York: Crown.

Lieberman, M. D., Inagaki, T. K., Tabibnia, G., & Crockett, M. J. (2011). Subjective responses to emotional stimuli during labeling, reappraisal, and distraction. *Emotion, 11*(3), 468–480.

Linehan, M. M., & Wilks, C. (2015). The course and evolution of dialectical behavior therapy. *American Journal of Psychotherapy, 69*(2), 97–110.

Lingiardi, V., & McWilliams, N. (Eds.). (2017). *Psychodynamic diagnostic manual* (2nd ed.): *PDM-2*. New York: Guilford Press.

Loewald, H. W. (1960). On the therapeutic action of psycho-analysis. *International Journal of Psychoanalysis, 41*, 16–33.

Loewald, H. W. (1970). Psychoanalytic theory and the psychoanalytic process. *Psychoanalytic Study of the Child, 25*, 45–68.

Loewenstein, G. (2007). Affect regulation and affective forecasting. In J. J. Gross (Ed.), *Handbook of emotion regulation* (pp. 180–203). New York: Guilford Press.

Lombardo, M. V., Chakrabarti, B., & Baron-Cohen, S. (2009). What neuroimaging and perceptions of self–other similarity can tell us about the mechanism underlying mentalizing. *Behavioral and Brain Sciences, 32*(2), 152–153.

Luyten, P., & Fonagy, P. (2015). The neurobiology of mentalizing. *Personality Disorders: Theory, Research, and Treatment, 6*(4), 366–379.

Luyten, P., van Houdenhove, B., Lemma, A., Target, M., & Fonagy, P. (2012). Vulnerability for functional somatic disorders: A contemporary psychodynamic approach. *Journal of Psychotherapy Integration, 23*(3), 250–262.

MacLeod, C., & Bucks, R. S. (2011). Emotion regulation and the cognitive-experimental approach to emotional dysfunction. *Emotion Review, 3*(1), 62–73.

Mahr, J., & Csibra, G. (2017). Why do we remember?: The communicative function of episodic memory. *Behavioral and Brain Sciences.* [Epub ahead of print]

Malcolm, J. (1981). *Psychoanalysis: The impossible profession.* New York: Knopf.

Malcolm, J. (1984). *In the Freud archives.* New York: Knopf.

Manguel, A. (2015). *Curiosity.* New Haven, CT: Yale University Press.

Markus, H. R., & Kitayama, S. (1991). Culture and the self: Implications for cognition, emotion, and motivation. *Psychological Review, 98*(2), 224–253.

Marty, P., & de M'Uzan, M. (1963). La pensée opératoire [Mentalization and action-bound thinking]. *Revue française de psychanalyse, 37*(22), 345–356. (Reprinted 1994 in *Revue française de psychosomatique, 6,* 197–207)

Marty, P., & Leighton, S. (2010). The narcissistic difficulties presented to the observer by the psychosomatic problem. *International Journal of Psychoanalysis, 91*(2), 347–363.

Mattila, A. K., Kronholm, E., Jula, A., Salminen, J. K., Koivisto, A., Mielonen, R., et al. (2008). Alexithymia and somatization in general population. *Psychosomatic Medicine, 70*(6), 716–722.

Mayer, J. D., & Salovey, P. (1997). What is emotional intelligence? In P. Salovey & D. J. Sluyter (Eds.), *Emotional development and emotional intelligence: Educational implications* (pp. 3–34). New York: Basic Books.

McDougall, J. (1989). *Theaters of the body: A psychoanalytic approach to psychosomatic illness.* New York: Norton.

McFall, R. M., Treat, T. A., & Simons, R. F. (2015). Clinical science model. In R. L. Cautin & S. O. Lillienfeld (Eds.), *The encyclopedia of clinical psychology* (pp. 1–9). Hoboken, NJ: Wiley.

McWilliams, N. (2011). *Psychoanalytic diagnosis: Understanding personality structure in the clinical process.* New York: Guilford Press.

Mennin, D. S., & Fresco, D. M. (2009). Emotion regulation as an integrative framework for understanding and treating psychopathology. In A. M. Kring & D. M. Sloan (Eds.), *Emotion regulation and psychopathology: A transdiagnostic approach to etiology and treatment* (pp. 356–379). New York: Guilford Press.

Mercier, H., & Sperber, D. (2011). Why do humans reason: Arguments for an argumentative theory. *Behavioral and Brain Sciences, 34,* 57–111.

Mitchell, P., Currie, G., & Ziegler, F. (2009). Two routes to perspective: Simulation and rule-use as approaches to mentalizing. *British Journal of Developmental Psychology, 27*(3), 515–543.

Mitchell, S. A. (1988). *Changing concepts of the analytic process: A method in search of new meanings.* Paper presented at the Relational Colloquium of the New York University Postdoctoral Program in Psychoanalysis, New York.

Moscovitch, M. (2012). The contribution of research on autobiographical memory to past and present theories of memory consolidation. In D. Berntsen & D. C. Rubin (Eds.), *Understanding autobiographical memory: Theories and approaches* (pp. 91–113). New York: Cambridge University Press.

Moscovitz, S. (2014). Hans Loewald's "On the therapeutic action of psychoanalysis": Initial reception and later influence. *Psychoanalytic Psychology, 31*(4), 575–587.

National Institute of Mental Health, U.S. Department of Health and Human Services. (2013, May 13). DSM-5 and RDoC: Shared interests [Press release]. Available from *www.nimh.nih.gov/news/science-news/2013/dsm-5-and-rdoc-shared-interests.shtml*.

Nelson, K., & Fivush, R. (2004). The emergence of autobiographical memory: A social cultural developmental theory. *Psychological Review, 111*(2), 486–511.

Nichols, S., & Stich, S. P. (2003). *Mindreading: An integrated account of pretence, self-awareness, and understanding other minds.* New York: Clarendon Press.

Ogden, T. H. (2015). Intuiting the truth of what's happening: On Bion's "'Notes on memory and desire." *Psychoanalytic Quarterly, 84*(2), 285–306.

Ogden, T. H. (2016). On language and truth in psychoanalysis. *Psychoanalytic Quarterly, 85*(2), 411–426.

Onishi, K. H., & Baillargeon, R. (2005). Do 15-month-old infants understand false beliefs? *Science, 308*(5719), 255–258.

Otis, L. (2015). *Rethinking thought: Inside the minds of creative scientists and artists.* New York: Oxford University Press.

Panksepp, J. (1998). *Affective neuroscience: The foundations of human and animal emotions.* New York: Oxford University Press.

Panksepp, J., & Biven, L. (2012). *The archaeology of mind: Neuroevolutionary origins of human emotions.* New York: Norton.

Pasupathi, M. (2003). Emotion regulation during social remembering: Differences between emotions elicited during an event and emotions elicited when talking about it. *Memory, 11*(2), 151–163.

Peirce, C. S. (1897). *Fallibilism, continuity, and evolution.* In C. Hartshorne & P. Weiss (Eds.), *Collected papers of Charles Sanders Peirce* (Vol. 1, pp. 141–175). Cambridge, MA: Harvard University Press.

Pennebaker, J. W. (1997). Writing about emotional experiences as a therapeutic process. *Psychological Science, 8*(3), 162–166.

Pessoa, L. (2008). On the relationship between emotion and cognition. *Nature Reviews Neuroscience, 9*(2), 148–158.

Philippe, F. L., Koestner, R., Lecours, S., Beaulieu-Pelletier, G., & Bois, K. (2011). The role of autobiographical memory networks in the experience of negative emotions: How our remembered past elicts our current feelings. *Emotion, 11*(6), 1279–1290.

Philippot, P., Baeyens, C., & Douilliez, C. (2006). Specifying emotional information: Regulation of emotional intensity via executive processes. *Emotion, 6*(4), 560–571.

Pillemer, D. B., & Kuwabara, K. J. (2012). Directive functions of autobiographical memory: Theory and method. In D. Berntsen & D. C. Rubin (Eds.), *Understanding autobiographical memory: Theories and approaches* (pp. 181–201). New York: Cambridge University Press.

Prebble, S. C., Addis, D. R., & Tippett, L. J. (2013). Autobiographical memory and sense of self. *Psychological Bulletin, 139*(4), 815–840.

Reber, R. (2016). *Critical feeling: How to use feelings strategically.* Cambridge, UK: Cambridge University Press.

Riding. A. (2007). Face to face with a life of creation. In R. Shargel (Ed.), *Ingmar Bergman interviews* (pp. 183–189). Jackson: University of Mississippi Press.

Rogers, A. (2017, May 11). Star neurologist Tom Insel leaves the Google-spawned verily for . . . A start up? *Wired.* Available at *www.wired.com/2017/05/star-neuroscientist-tom-insel-leaves-google-spawned-verily-startup.*

Rubin, D. C. (2012). The basic systems model of autobiographical memory. In D. Berntsen & D. C. Rubin (Eds.), *Understanding autobiographical memory: Theories and approaches* (pp. 11–32). New York: Cambridge University Press.

Russell, J. A. (1991). Culture and the categorization of emotions. *Psychological Bulletin, 110*(3), 426–450.

Sacks, O. (1998). *The man who mistook his wife for a hat and other clinical tales.* New York: Touchstone.

Sacks, O. (2001). *Uncle tungsten: Memories of a chemical boyhood.* New York: Knopf.

Sacks, O. (2010, December 31). This year, change your mind. *New York Times.* Available from *www.nytimes.com/2011/01/01/opinion/01sacks.html.*

Sacks, O. (2013, July 6). The joy of old age. (No kidding.) *New York Times.* Available from *www.nytimes.com/2013/07/07/opinion/sunday/the-joy-of-old-age-no-kidding.html.*

Sacks, O. (2015, June 5a). Mishearings. *New York Times.* Available from *www.nytimes.com/2015/06/07/opinion/oliver-sacks-mishearings.html.*

Sacks, O. (2015b, February 19). My own life: Oliver Sacks on learning he has terminal cancer. *New York Times.* Available from *www.nytimes.com/2015/02/19/opinion/oliver-sacks-on-learning-he-has-terminal-cancer.html.*

Sacks, O. (2015c, July 24). Oliver Sacks: My periodic table. *New York Times.* Available from *www.nytimes.com/2015/07/26/opinion/my-periodic-table.html.*

Sacks, O. (2015d, August 14). Oliver Sacks: Sabbath. *New York Times.* Available from *www.nytimes.com/2015/08/16/opinion/sunday/oliver-sacks-sabbath.html.*

Sacks, O. (2015e). *On the move: A life.* New York: Knopf.

Sacks, O. (2016). *Gratitude.* New York: Knopf.

Safran, J. (2012). Doublethinking or dialectical thinking: A critical appreciation of Hoffman's "doublethinking" critique. *Psychoanalytic Dialogues, 22,* 710–720.

Schall, M., Martiny, S. E., Goetz, T., & Hall, N. C. (2016). Smiling on the inside: The social benefits of suppressing positive emotions in outperformance situations. *Personality and Social Psychology Bulletin, 42*(5), 559–571.

Scheidt, C. E., Waller, E., Schnock, C., Becker-Stoll, F., Zimmermann, P., Lücking, C. H., et al. (1999). Alexithymia and attachment representation in idiopathic Spasmodic Torticollis. *Journal of Nervous and Mental Disease, 187*(1), 47–52.

Schore, A. N. (1994). *Affect regulation and the origin of the self: The neurobiology of emotional development.* Hillsdale, NJ: Erlbaum.

Schore, A. N. (2003). *Affect regulation and the repair of the self.* New York: Norton.

Schutte, N. S., Malouff, J. M., Hall, L. E., Haggerty, D. J., Cooper, J. T., Golden, C. J., et al. (1998). Development and validation of a measure of emotional intelligence. *Personality and Individual Differences, 25*(2), 167–177.

Selcuk, E., Zayas, V., Günaydin, G., Hazan, C., & Kross, E. (2012). Mental representations of attachment figures facilitate recovery following upsetting autobiographical memory recall. *Journal of Personality and Social Psychology, 103*(2), 362–378.

Shanton, K., & Goldman, A. (2010). Simulation theory. *Wiley Interdisciplinary Reviews: Cognitive Science, 1*(4), 527–538.

Shapiro, S. L., Carlson, L. E., Astin, J. A., & Freedman, B. (2006). Mechanisms of mindfulness. *Journal of Clinical Psychology, 62*(3), 373–386.

Sharp, C., & Venta, A. (2012). Mentalizing problems in children and adolescents. In N. Midgley & I. Vrouva (Eds.), *Minding the child: Mentalization-based interventions with children, young people and their families* (pp. 35–53). New York: Routledge/Taylor & Francis.

Shay, J. (2014). Moral injury. *Psychoanalytic Psychology, 31*(2), 182–191.

Shedler, J. (2010). The efficacy of psychodynamic psychotherapy. *American Psychologist, 65*(2), 98–109.

Sherman, N. (2014). Recovering lost goodness: Shame, guilt, and self-empathy. *Psychoanalytic Psychology, 31*(2), 217–235.

Shweder, R. (1994). "You're not sick, you're just in love": Emotion as an interpretive system. In P. Ekman & R. J. Davidson (Eds.), *The nature of emotions: Fundamental questions* (pp. 32–44). New York: Oxford University Press.

Siegel, D. J. (2007). *The mindful brain: Reflection and attunement in the cultivation of well-being.* New York: Norton.

Silverman, S. (2010). *The bedwetter: Stories of courage, redemption, and pee.* New York: Harper.

Smith, M. D. (2016). *Invisible man, got the whole world watching: A young black man's education.* New York: Nation Books.

Smith, T. K. (2011). *Life on mars: Poems.* Minneapolis, MN: Graywolf Press.

Smith, T. K. (2015). *Ordinary light: A memoir.* New York: Knopf.

Snow, C. P. (1959). *The two cultures and the scientific revolution.* New York: Cambridge University Press.

Solbakken, O. A., Hansen, R. S., Havik, O. E., & Monsen, J. T. (2011).

Assessment of affect integration: Validation of the affect consciousness construct. *Journal of Personality Assessment, 93*(3), 257–265.

Solbakken, O. A., Hansen, R. S., & Monsen, J. T. (2011). Affect integration and reflective function: Clarification of central conceptual issues. *Psychotherapy Research, 21*(4), 482–496.

Solomon, A. (2015, May 11). "On the move," by Oliver Sacks. *New York Times.* Available from *www.nytimes.com/2015/05/17/books/review/on-the-move-by-oliver-sacks.html?_r=0.*

Spence, D. P. (1982). *Narrative truth and historical truth: Meaning and interpretation in psychoanalysis.* New York: Norton.

Spence, D. P. (1983). Narrative persuasion. *Psychoanalysis and Contemporary Thought, 6*(3), 457–481.

Sperber, D., Clément, F., Heintz, C., Mascaro, O., Mercier, H., Origgi, G., et al. (2010). Epistemic vigilance. *Mind and Language, 25*(4), 359–393.

Spezzano, C. (1993). *Affect in psychoanalysis: A clinical synthesis.* London: Routledge.

Steele, H. (2013). Perspective 5: Earliest experiences and attachment processes. In D. Narvaez, J. Panksepp, A. N. Schore, & T. R. Gleason (Eds.), *Evolution, early experience and human development: From research to practice and policy* (pp. 421–426). New York: Oxford University Press.

Steele, H., & Steele, M. (2008). On the origins of reflective functioning. In F. N. Busch (Ed.), *Mentalization: Theoretical considerations, research findings, and clinical implications* (pp. 133–158). New York: Analytic Press.

Stern, D. B. (2013a). Field theory in psychoanalysis: Part 1. Harry Stack Sullivan and Madeleine and Willy Baranger. *Psychoanalytic Dialogues, 23*(5), 487–501.

Stern, D. B. (2013b). Field theory in psychoanalysis: Part 2. Bionian field theory and contemporary interpersonal/relational psychoanalysis. *Psychoanalytic Dialogues, 23*(6), 630–645.

Stern, D. N. (1985). *The interpersonal world of the infant: A view from psychoanalysis and developmental psychology.* New York: Basic Books.

Strenger, C. (2013). Why psychoanalysis must not discard science and human nature. *Psychoanalytic Dialogues, 23*(2), 197–210.

Stueber, K. (2006). *Rediscovering empathy: Agency, folk psychology, and the human sciences.* Cambridge, MA: MIT Press.

Summers, F. (2013). *The psychoanalytic vision: The experiencing subject, transcendence, and the therapeutic process.* New York: Routledge/Taylor & Francis.

Suri, G., Whittaker, K., & Gross, J. J. (2015). Launching reappraisal: It's less common than you might think. *Emotion, 15*(1), 73–77.

Sutin, A. R., & Gillath, O. (2009). Autobiographical memory phenomenology and content mediate attachment style and psychological distress. *Journal of Counseling Psychology, 56*(3), 351–364.

Taubner, S., Hörg, S., Fischer-Stern, M., Doering, S., Buckheim, A., & Zimmerman, J. (2013). Internal structure of the reflective functioning scale. *Psychological Assessment, 25*(1), 127–135.

Taylor, G. J., & Bagby, R. M. (2013). Psychoanalysis and empirical research: The example of alexithymia. *Journal of the American Psychoanalytic Association, 61*(1), 99–133.

Taylor, G. J., Bagby, R. M., & Parker, J. D. (1997). *Disorders of affect regulation: Alexithymia in medical and psychiatric illness.* Cambridge, UK: Cambridge University Press.

Tomasello, M. (2016). Cultural learning redux. *Child Development, 87*(3), 643–653.

Tomkins, S. S. (1991). *Affect, imagery, consciousness: Vol. 3. The negative affects: Anger and fear.* New York: Springer.

Tomkins, S. S. (1995). *Shame and its sisters: A Silvan Tomkins reader* (K. Sedgwick, A. Frank, & I. E. Alexander, Eds.). Durham, NC: Duke University Press.

Tulving, E. (2005). Episodic memory and autonoesis: Uniquely human? In H. S. Terrace & J. Metcalfe (Eds.), *The missing link in cognition: Origins of self-reflective consciousness* (pp. 3–56). New York: Oxford University Press.

Turkle, S. (2015). *Reclaiming conversation: The power of talk in a digital age.* New York: Penguin Press.

Waters, S. F., Virmani, E. A., Thompson, R. A., Meyer, S., Raikes, H. A., & Jochem, R. (2010). Emotion regulation and attachment: Unpacking two constructs and their association. *Journal of Psychopathology and Behavioral Assessment, 32*(1), 37–47.

Webb, T. L., Miles, E., & Sheeran, P. (2012). Dealing with feeling: A meta-analysis of the effectiveness of strategies derived from the process model of emotion regulation. *Psychological Bulletin, 138*(4), 775–808.

Webber, R. (2016, January 5). Odd emotions. Available from *www.psychology-today.com/articles/201601/odd-emotions*.

Westphal, M., Seivert, N. H., & Bonanno, G. A. (2010). Expressive flexibility. *Emotion, 10*(1), 92–100.

Wheeler, M. A., Stuss, D. T., & Tulving, E. (1997). Toward a theory of episodic memory: The frontal lobes and autonoetic consciousness. *Psychological Bulletin, 121*(3), 331–354.

Wilkinson, M. R., & Ball, L. J. (2012). Why studies of autism spectrum disorders have failed to resolve the theory theory versus simulation theory debate. *Review of Philosophy and Psychology, 3*(2), 263–291.

Williams, B. (2002). *Truth and truthfulness: An essay in genealogy.* Princeton, NJ: Princeton University Press.

Williams, J. M. G., Barnhofer, T., Crane, C., Hermans, D., Raes, F., Watkins, E., et al. (2007). Autobiographical memory specificity and emotional disorder. *Psychological Bulletin, 133*(1), 122–148.

Winnicott, D. W. (1965). *The maturational processes and the facilitating environment: Studies in the theory of emotional development.* Oxford, UK: International Universities Press.

Winter, A. (2012). *Memory: Fragments of a modern history.* Chicago: University of Chicago Press.

Woolfolk, R. L. (2015). *The value of psychotherapy: The talking cure in an age of clinical science.* New York: Guilford Press.

Yadlin-Gadot, S. (2017) [Ef]facing truth: Between philosophy and psychoanalysis. *Journal of Theoretical and Philosophical Psychology, 37*(1), 1–20.

Yandoli, K.L. (2017, September 25). This video series featuring Sarah Silverman and Lena Dunham aims to destigmatize therapy. *BuzzFeed News*. Available at *www.buzzfeed.com/krystieyandoli/this-video-series-featuring-sarah-silverman-and-lena-dunham?utm_term=.fjOOVVXrZ#.lirW99P7X*.

Young, R. (1986). *Personal autonomy: Beyond negative and positive liberty.* London: Croom Helm.

Zaretsky, E. (2005). *Secrets of the soul: A social and cultural history of psychoanalysis.* New York: Vintage.

Index